S.E. WEAVER
905 MAIN AVE.
BROWNWOOD, TEXAS 76801

TOUCH, TASTE, SMELL, SIGHT AND HEARING

This volume is one of a series designed to familiarize readers
with the latest advances in medical science as a guide in
maintaining their own health and fitness.

TOUCH, TASTE, SMELL, SIGHT AND HEARING

by Wendy Murphy

AND THE EDITORS OF TIME-LIFE BOOKS

LIBRARY OF HEALTH / TIME-LIFE BOOKS / ALEXANDRIA, VIRGINIA

THE AUTHOR:
Wendy Murphy has written several volumes for Time-Life
Books, including *Coping with the Common Cold* and
Dealing with Headaches in the Library of Health, and two
volumes of the TIME-LIFE Encyclopedia of Gardening:
Japanese Gardening and *Indoor Gardening Under Light*. In
25 years of writing and editing, she has developed expertise
in a wide range of additional subjects, from antiques and
boating to paleontology and home repair.

THE CONSULTANTS:
Dr. Ralph Frederick Naunton has lectured and written
extensively on diseases of the ear and on techniques for the
detection and treatment of hearing loss. His books include
Modern Developments in Audiology and *An Introduction to
Audiometry*. A former president of the American Audiology
Society, he served for 12 years as head of the department of
otolaryngology at the University of Chicago.

Dr. Peter Y. Evans is Chairman of the Department
of Ophthalmology at the Georgetown University School of
Medicine in Washington, D.C., and Vice Chairman of
Ophthalmology at Sibley Memorial Hospital. He serves as a
senior consultant for the Veterans Administration Hospital,
and supervises eye care at the District Training School in
Laurel, Md. Dr. Evans has done research in strabismus and
won awards for his work in cineangiography, a method of
filming the eye's circulatory system in action.

For information about any Time-Life book, please write:
Reader Information, Time-Life Books,
541 North Fairbanks Court, Chicago, Illinois 60611.

First printing. Printed in U.S.A.
Published simultaneously in Canada.
School and library distribution by Silver Burdett
Company, Morristown, New Jersey.

TIME-LIFE is a trademark of Time Incorporated U.S.A.

Library of Congress Cataloguing in Publication Data
Murphy, Wendy B., 1935-
　　Touch, Smell, Taste, Sight and Hearing
　　(Library of Health)
　　Bibliography: p.
　　Includes index.
　　1. Senses and sensation.　　2. Sense organs—
Diseases.
　　I. Time-Life Books.　II. Title.　III. Series.
QP431.M78　　　　612.8　　　82-5738
ISBN 0-8094-3800-3　　　　AACR2
ISBN 0-8094-3799-6 (lib. bdg.)
ISBN 0-8094-3798-8 (ret. ed.)

Time-Life Books Inc. is a wholly owned subsidiary of
TIME INCORPORATED

FOUNDER: Henry R. Luce 1898-1967

Editor-in-Chief: Henry Anatole Grunwald
President: J. Richard Munro
Chairman of the Board: Ralph P. Davidson
Executive Vice President: Clifford J. Grum
Chairman, Executive Committee: James R. Shepley
Editorial Director: Ralph Graves
Group Vice President, Books: Joan D. Manley
Vice Chairman: Arthur Temple

TIME-LIFE BOOKS INC.

EDITOR: George Constable
Director of Design: Louis Klein
Executive Editor: George Daniels
Board of Editors: Dale M. Brown, Thomas H. Flaherty Jr., William Frankel,
Thomas A. Lewis, Martin Mann, John Paul Porter, Gerry
Schremp, Gerald Simons, Kit van Tulleken
Director of Administration: David L. Harrison
Director of Research: Carolyn L. Sackett
Director of Photography: Dolores Allen Littles

President: Carl G. Jaeger
Executive Vice Presidents: John Steven Maxwell, David J. Walsh
Vice Presidents: George Artandi, Stephen L. Bair, Peter G. Barnes,
Nicholas Benton, John L. Canova, Beatrice T. Dobie,
James L. Mercer

LIBRARY OF HEALTH

Editors: Martin Mann, William Frankel
Designer: Albert Sherman
Chief Researcher: Jo Thomson
Editorial Staff for *Touch, Smell, Taste, Sight and Hearing*
Picture Editor: Jane Speicher Jordan
Text Editors: Tyler Mathisen, Brian McGinn, Donia Whiteley Mills
Writers: Deborah Berger-Turnbull, William deLaunay Worsley
Researchers: Norma E. Kennedy, Sara Mark (principals),
Jean B. Crawford, Judy D. French, Jonn Ethan Hankins,
Sheirazada Hann, Patricia N. McKinney
Assistant Designers: Anne K. DuVivier, Cynthia T. Richardson
Copy Coordinators: Margery duMond, Stephen G. Hyslop
Picture Coordinator: Rebecca C. Christoffersen
Editorial Assistant: Margaret A. Zank
Special Contributors: Christopher S. Conner, Phyllis E. Lehmann, Lydia Preston,
Dr. Edward L. Zimney (writers); Barbara Lerner (researcher)

EDITORIAL OPERATIONS
Production Director: Feliciano Madrid
Assistant: Peter A. Inchauteguiz
Copy Processing: Gordon E. Buck
Quality Control Director: Robert L. Young
Assistant: James J. Cox
Associates: Daniel J. McSweeney, Michael G. Wight
Art Coordinator: Anne B. Landry
Copy Room Director: Susan Galloway Goldberg
Assistants: Celia Beattie, Ricki Tarlow

Correspondents: Elisabeth Kraemer (Bonn); Margot
Hapgood, Dorothy Bacon (London); Susan Jonas, Lucy T.
Voulgaris (New York); Maria Vincenza Aloisi, Josephine du
Brusle (Paris); Ann Natanson (Rome).
Valuable assistance was also provided by: Judy Aspinall
(London); John Dunn (Melbourne); Miriam Hsia (New York).

CONTENTS

CHAPTER 1

Five ways to grasp the world

Mysteries of touch
Reading the complex language of odors
A feast of tastes from sweet, salt, sour and bitter
Why people see better than animals
Hearing: the sense that is always turned on

At the outset of *Remembrance of Things Past,* the master-work of French novelist Marcel Proust, the narrator nibbles a madeleine—a sweet, shell-shaped wafer—soaked in tea, savoring its taste and aroma. Suddenly, magically, the doors of memory swing open; the narrator is transported back to the same experience in his childhood, to the sights and sounds of his family's garden and eventually to a host of memories and associations that come to fill the 16 volumes of the novel. All of this from a cookie and a cup of tea—yet the experience is of a kind that everyone has known. The impressions of such senses as taste and smell, which often seem fragile and ephemeral, turn out to be powerful and unforgettable.

What is more, a constant stream of new perceptions turns out to be indispensable to human life. How indispensable the senses are becomes clear when they are missing. Since the 1950s, scientists have conducted experiments in which volunteers are deprived of all sensation. In the simplest of these tests, subjects are placed in a soundproofed, pitch-black room, their hands gloved to blunt the sense of touch. In others they are floated completely submersed in tepid water, breathing filtered, odor-free air through a mask. Sight, hearing, smell, taste, touch—even the subtle sense that records the pull of gravity upon the body—are utterly blanked out.

The results of these experiments are astonishing. Lack of sensation has devastating impact. Few subjects can endure it more than six hours. Cut off from the outside world, they

succumb to tension and anxiety. Fantasies and hallucinations fill the mind. The subjects soon lose their capacity for concentration and for organized, logical thought. Fortunately, these losses are temporary, but they point to a function of the senses that was never before fully realized. In the words of psychiatrists Philip Solomon and Susan Kleeman of the University of California: "Even man's conscious mind can now be seen to be intimately dependent on continuous changing stimuli from the outside world. Variety is the spice, even the staff, of life."

Although each of the senses seems unique—the feel of a piece of velvet apparently unrelated to the smell of a rose or the glare of a bright light—a deep unity of anatomy and nerve processes links them all. Each sense receives information from the external world by means of nerve cells called receptors, lying on or just beneath the surface of the body. In turn each of these sets of passive sensors is linked by a network of nerves to a part of the brain designed to interpret the information *(page 25)*.

The receptors for each sense are stimulated by one particular kind of energy—mechanical energy for touch and hearing, chemical energy for smell and taste, radiant energy for sight. By a process called transduction, the receptors for each sense convert that received energy into a language of electrical impulses. Sometimes, as in the skin, this occurs instantaneously; sometimes, as in the ear, at the end of a Rube Goldberg string of living hardware. It is in this transduced form of energy, a kind of internal Morse code, that all senso-

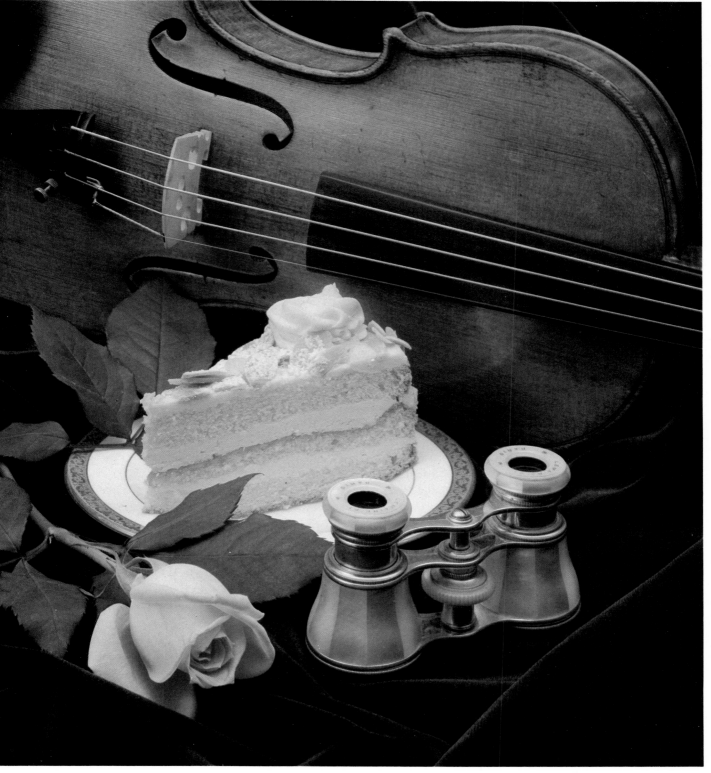

The human senses, providing integrated powers of perception superior to those of any other creature, bring to the brain the delights of music, the softness of velvet, the taste of cake, the aroma of roses and the spectacle of the world. More important, the nerve signals enable people to avoid danger, do work and, in a supremely human achievement, communicate with their fellows.

ry information travels along the nerve pathways to the brain.

Because all of the senses are basic to survival and all of them contribute to the quality of life, the loss or impairment of any of these is potentially devastating. Even a slight deterioration is a real loss: The constant smoker who muffles his sense of smell loses some of the pleasure and benefits of food. Understanding the senses, safeguarding them, and easing or curing their disorders are essential elements of good health care.

Mysteries of touch

In the Fourth Century B.C., Aristotle, the great scientific classifier of ancient Greece, worked out a view of the senses as five separate systems. When he came to touch, however, he hesitated. "It is a problem," he wrote, "whether touch is a single sense or a group of senses."

He had good reason to be puzzled. What Aristotle chose to call touch turns out to be a complex cluster of skin-deep senses, reporting not only contact and pressure, but also heat, cold and pain. Deep within the body, a related sense sends the brain signals of pressure and pain—the pain of inflamed tissue in arthritis, for example, or of swollen blood vessels in a headache. Still other signals, coming from every part of the body, give the brain information about the positions of muscles, bones and limbs.

To the conscious mind, the sense of touch residing at or near the skin is most important, because it ceaselessly gathers information from the outside world. But the skin itself is not an organ, comparable to the tongue, nose, eye or ear. Like the heart or the liver, these sense organs are assemblies of tissue adapted to perform a specific function. For the sense of touch, specialized receptors are distributed all over the skin, each adapted to detect a particular form or state of contact, pressure, temperature or pain.

No fewer than seven anatomical types of such receptors have so far been identified *(pages 26-27)*, and the list is still far from complete. Some of the gaps are tantalizing: Though the receptor for cold, to take one example, is now known, the corresponding one for warmth—which must exist—has yet to be identified. Nevertheless, the task of mapping the loca-

tions of both known and unknown receptors by triggering their sensations has been performed with much precision.

It appears that virtually all surface areas of the body contain every kind of touch receptor, but in different numbers and densities. To map them, researchers systematically study every area of the skin for typical patterns of sensitivity and discrimination. For example, in a standard procedure called a two-point discrimination test, the scientists use pairs of pins, feathers and other instruments. The tips of each pair of probes are set at varying distances from one another and applied to the skin; for each setting, subjects report whether they feel two probes or one.

Discrimination varies enormously from one part of the skin to another. Most discriminating of all are the tongue— an infant's first major tool of sensory exploration—and the fingertips, with which a blind person reads braille, a magician does sleight of hand and a safecracker feels the movement of tumblers in a lock. At the tip of the tongue, the tips of probes are sensed as separate points when they are only $\frac{1}{25}$ inch apart; on the fingertip, when they are $\frac{1}{10}$ inch apart. Running a close third are the lips and the tip of the nose; these areas are sufficiently rich in receptors to feel probe tips $\frac{1}{4}$ inch apart. From these high levels, discrimination falls off sharply. At the front of the torso the probe tips are not felt as two separate points of pressure until they are $1\frac{1}{2}$ inches apart; at the center of the back they must be 3 inches apart.

Most touch sensations tend to fade rather quickly; nerve endings become relatively insensitive to constant, unchanging stimulation in a matter of seconds. Clothes, for example, elicit sensations when you put them on in the morning; thereafter, except for moments when you move and the clothes rub your body, the sense of touch scarcely takes notice of them. In the same way, the pressure felt when you sit down in a chair or lean against a wall is soon forgotten, and a hot bath no longer seems hot. Only when a new event occurs—perhaps the landing of a fly on the skin—is a sensation felt.

On a larger scale, touching and being touched play a key role in the development of the other senses, and in an infant's physical growth. In the 1940s, American psychiatrist Marga-

THE TENDER PLACES

Sensitivity to pressure varies greatly over the body; it is most acute at the delicate tip of the tongue, and least so on the ball of the foot. The relative responsiveness of nine points on the body are indicated by color on the figure at right and identified in the list below, which names them in descending order of sensitivity.

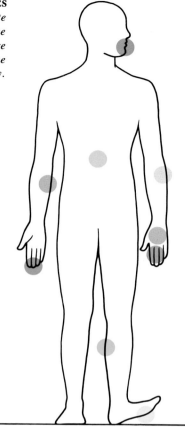

TIP OF TONGUE
TIP OF FINGER
BACK OF FINGER
INSIDE OF FOREARM
BACK OF HAND
CALF
ABDOMEN
OUTSIDE OF FOREARM
SOLE

ret A. Ribble found that increased handling of infants stimulated their respiration and blood flow, and more recent research has shown that touch sensations are a kind of dress rehearsal for the mastery of more complex sensory skills, such as seeing and hearing.

At birth, an infant has the basic equipment for recording and associating sensory impressions, but for most of the senses, this equipment is not yet fully formed. Only the sense of touch is primed and ready to go immediately. From the moment of birth the child begins to communicate with parents by physical contact. As fingers, toes, and mouth are pressed into service, the baby becomes aware of both his own body and the outside world of textures, shapes and temperatures. According to psychologist Donald O. Hebb of McGill University, each tactile experience strengthens a rudimentary nerve pathway to the brain, gradually creating an organized network. Upon this foundation—in Hebb's view—rises the scaffolding of later learning.

If touching babies is good for them, failing to touch them is bad—very bad. The facts have long been known, largely through studies of children in orphanages. In 1915 a survey of foundling homes in the United States showed that, in nine out of 10 of these institutions, the death rate for infants under one year of age was nearly 100 per cent. Cleanliness and nutrition had little or no bearing on how the children fared; almost routinely, they developed a disease called marasmus (from a Greek word for "dying away"), marked by loss of appetite, listlessness and the atrophy of the body.

A Boston physician, Dr. Fritz Talbot, was probably the first American to realize that lack of handling was a principal cause of the mysterious ailment. Reporting on his discovery, he described a pre-World War I visit to the Children's Clinic in Düsseldorf, Germany. Walking around the wards with the Clinic's director, Dr. Arthur Schlossmann, he was impressed with the tidiness of the place, but then he noticed something that seemed curiously out of place. A fat old woman who did not appear to be part of the staff was walking the corridor with a puny child on her hip. "Who's that?" he asked the director. "Oh, that," replied Dr. Schlossmann, "is Old Anna. When we have done everything we can medically for a

baby, and it is still not doing well, we turn it over to Old Anna, and she is always successful."

Dr. Talbot reasoned that Old Anna was providing something all children need to thrive and develop: holding and cuddling, or as he expressed it, in a phrase that has become a permanent fixture of American English, "tender loving care." TLC programs were gradually implemented in American children's institutions of many kinds. Even in hospitals, where the level of health care was already high, the programs produced astonishing results. At New York's Bellevue Hospital, for example, nurses in the pediatric wards began a daily routine in which each child was regularly held and stroked; the mortality rates for infants under one year fell from 35 per cent to less than 10 per cent.

Aside from this crucial role during infancy, the sense of touch is not an aspect of health that most people think about. At any age, however, a person who experiences a disorder of touch sensations, however mild, should consult a physician. Although such disorders are usually trivial and temporary, the possibility of serious disease is real enough to warrant investigation. Neuritis and neuralgia, for example, can cause the skin and underlying area to suffer sensations of ''pins and needles'' and occasional stabbing pain with little or no apparent stimulation. Numbness may be a warning symptom of stroke, brain tumor or a lesion on the spinal cord. Excruciating pain in the hands and feet may accompany the viral disease called shingles.

Even when an underlying disease is successfully treated, normal sensory function may not be fully restored. Because touch involves diffuse nerve endings and a vast network of nerve fibers, its failures are difficult to deal with. When the problem is one of permanent pain, as in some cases of neuralgia, the remedy may involve cutting the nerves that carry the pain—which may leave the patient with a new set of handicaps, such as numbness and even paralysis.

Reading the complex language of odors

While the sense of touch is spread through all of the skin, that of smell resides in a single organ. A 16th Century Italian man of letters, Stefano Guazzo, was certain he knew the reason for the location of that organ. ''The nose,'' he wrote, ''is placed above the mouth to this end, that all those things wherewith we feed our bellies must first pay tribute to the nose, and from thence have their passport and assurance for nourishment in our bellies.''

The idea almost buried in Guazzo's imagery is sound as far as it goes, but it does not go far enough. A nose does gather information about food as the food is eaten, and its strategic position just above the mouth is perfect for the job of approving or rejecting whatever passes by. Most of the time, however, the nose scans nonfood odors from the surrounding air. It does so with amazing sensitivity and precision, mainly as a protection against danger—warning of noxious gases, for example. In addition, the sense of smell influences animal and human behavior in some previously unsuspected ways.

Odors are made up of molecules that diffuse through air and are carried long distances by wind. Their use by animals in hunting prey or detecting predators has long been known, but only in recent decades has the extent of their importance been understood. A class of odorous substances called pheromones, generated in the normal course of life, serve as biological activators. In moths, a pheromone secreted by a gland in the female can attract a male moth half a mile away; a single female can produce enough at one time to attract a billion males. In beehives and anthills pheromones carry signals for alarm and attack, grooming and food gathering. Mother seals find their own young by scent in a breeding ground filled with thousands of apparently identical pups.

Pheromones may have a role in human society, too. In 1971, Harvard psychologist Martha McClintock noted that women students who were roommates tended to synchronize their menstrual periods to a far greater degree than random pairs of women. Soon afterward, Michael Russel at San Francisco State University directly linked menstrual synchronization to the sense of smell. Three times a week, Russel daubed the upper lips of a group of female subjects with a solution containing drops of perspiration from one woman—an individual unacquainted with the test subjects. Within four months their menstrual cycles swung drastically to conform with hers.

In themselves, such experiments show little more than the fact that pheromones are generated and perceived in human beings as well as animals. But the study of human pheromones is still in its infancy; these substances may prove to have something like the range and power of their animal counterparts, and thus to regulate many functions of the human body by odors. Meanwhile, although the mechanisms of regulation remain mysterious, the process by which the odors are detected is pretty well understood. Every odor—of a pheromone, a rose, a skunk or whatever—is sensed in the same way and by the same organ.

That organ is not strictly the nose. The true organ of smell consists of a pair of yellow-brown, mucus-covered patches, the olfactory membranes, each about the area of a dime, and both tucked into a cul de sac at the very top of the nasal cavity, behind and slightly above the bridge of the nose. Within the membranes are olfactory cells, equipped with hairlike antennae that project through the protective blanket of mucus to scan the passing air stream.

The sensation of smell, essentially a chemical stimulation, occurs as a by-product of breathing. A breath of inhaled air contains trillions of molecules. An overwhelming majority are molecules of two odorless gases, nitrogen and oxygen, but dispersed among them are molecules of odorous substances, which can be sensed in infinitesimal quantities. The chemical that carries the defensive odor of a skunk, for example, is perceived if a person inhales a mere 19 million molecules—or .000000000000071 ounce.

In normal breathing only a tiny fraction of inhaled air comes into contact with the olfactory membranes; while the mainstream of a breath takes the low road to the throat and lungs, tiny eddies float upward to the olfactory membrane. To take a larger sample, the nose sniffs, altering the air flow so that a larger share of the air stream is forced upward. And to monitor food as it is eaten, the nose uses particles, released in chewing and swallowing, that rise from the back of the mouth to the nasal cavity and waft over the olfactory patches.

Contact between an odor-producing molecule and an olfactory antenna starts a sequence of terse neural communications: The olfactory nerve cell fires an electrical message to the olfactory bulb, a collecting station just below the brain, and the bulb in turn signals the brain itself. Many details of the process remain unclear. No one has been able to give an entirely satisfactory explanation of how the olfactory apparatus distinguishes one smell from another—yet distinguish it does, and superbly. In one of Sir Arthur Conan Doyle's tales, Sherlock Holmes notes that a good detective should be able to identify at least 75 smells. In fact, ordinary mortals regularly discern thousands of different odors.

The ability to discern odors is not the same as an ability to identify the substances that produce them. According to psychologist William S. Cain of Yale University, a typical subject in a blindfold test of 80 familiar odors generally thinks he knows all of them but can name no more than 36 correctly. With practice, almost anyone can improve the score enormously; some subjects identify as many as 75 of the 80 substances after only five trials.

Women, who tend to do better on such tests, also tend to use a more varied vocabulary in describing the smells, and

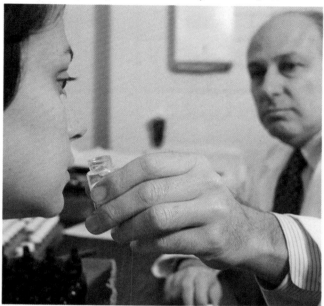

Testing a patient whose sense of smell is impaired, Dr. Robert I. Henkin asks her to identify a banana-scented solution; knowing which odors she cannot recognize may indicate the cause of the sensory loss. Causes may range from head injury to dietary deficiency. One controversial theory, supported by Dr. Henkin, blames some olfactory loss on an inability to absorb zinc.

the ability to label smells seems to help in remembering familiar odors. Certainly, standardized naming systems help professionals in such businesses as perfume manufacturing, brewing and winemaking. The American Society of Brewing Chemists, for example, recognizes nine general aroma categories and 33 specific odors that may be found in beer. By labeling selected batches—"too hoppy," "too nutty," "too papery," "not malty enough"—the brewmasters maintain a standard flavor.

While some scientists trace the diversity of odors, others have tried to discover a basic system of sensory building blocks by which to organize them—a system comparable to the primary colors, which combine to produce an almost infinite variety of tints. The Greek philosopher Plato simply placed all odors in two classes: pleasant and unpleasant. His student Aristotle named six—sweet, bitter, pungent, astringent, acid and succulent. The 18th Century scientist Linnaeus had his own list: aromatic, fragrant, musky, garlicky, goaty, repulsive and nauseous.

The listmaking continues; many physiologists are now

convinced that all smells, however elusive, are reducible to primaries. The search for these primaries was influenced by the Scottish chemist R. W. Moncrieff, who suggested in the late 1940s that the geometric shapes of molecules determine the smell sensations they elicit. Specific molecular shapes, Moncrieff argued, fit the surface terrains of specific receptors in the olfactory membranes.

In 1962 biochemist John E. Amoore applied Moncrieff's hypothesis to develop a new classification system. Amoore proposed a list of seven odor primaries: camphoraceous (like mothballs), musky, floral, pepperminty, ethereal (etherlike), pungent, and putrid. By 1964, he and his associates at Georgetown University in Washington, D.C., had laid out a theory of the mechanism of odor discrimination. Their proposal followed Moncrieff's idea in describing the first five primaries. These, they proposed, are produced by molecules with shapes that fit into corresponding receptors like keys into a lock. Pungent and putrid odors work differently; it is not the shape but the fact that their molecules carry distinctive electrical charges that creates the fit. Molecules with pungent odors carry a positive charge; those with putrid, a negative. Both presumably cling to receptors of an opposite electrical charge.

In this maze of research and speculation, Plato's old categories of pleasant and unpleasant odors are almost forgotten. Most people might be expected to agree that some of Amoore's categories—floral and pepperminty, for example—are pleasant; others, such as putrid, are generally considered unpleasant. But culture, heredity and age produce differences of perception. Most Mediterranean people delight in the odor of garlic; many Northern Europeans, raised on a garlic-free diet, abhor the smell. The untutored American nose often rejects a host of exotic spices, "fishy-smelling" fish and aged cheeses that are prized as olfactory delicacies elsewhere.

Genetic influences can affect the sense of smell more violently and completely. For example, failures of the olfactory sense may arise in hereditary disorders of the nervous system, or in equally hereditary endocrine disorders that subtly distort body chemistry. The malfunction may show up in members of the same family; in some families, everyone is odor-blind to one or a few substances.

Such disorders do not generally create a handicap comparable to the loss of touch, but they are more than a mere inconvenience, as indicated by the case of a patient who consulted Dr. Ralph Naunton at the National Institutes of Health. "The young lady was in her mid-twenties when I met her," Dr. Naunton later recalled. "Born without a sense of smell, she had fared reasonably well as long as she was living at home with her parents, but now she was in a place of her own and having a devil of a time.

"Whenever her mother visited her, the young woman was gently rebuked for rancid smells in her refrigerator. When she tried preparing dinner for a beau, the food was either underseasoned or overseasoned. Perfume went on with about the same degree of success. Without someone sniffing over her shoulder all the time, she worried whether her breath, her body and her bathroom smelled sweet. What was far worse, she had nightmares that smoke, a gas leak, spoiled food, toxic chemicals—things that most people are alerted to by their identifying smells—would someday do her in."

Dr. Naunton tested the woman in the hope of finding some simple medical problem, simply remedied. There was none. "I had to tell her that, unfortunately, there was nothing medically we could do for her. Her only recourse, short of going home again, was to be obsessively fastidious in her person and her housekeeping, to learn to cook with the precision of a lab technician, and to get a roommate."

Age can bring on smell disorders, particularly after the body's metabolic processes slow down. Though olfactory receptors renew themselves, they do so at the rate of once every 30 days—about one third the renewal rate of taste buds. Both rates slow progressively during middle age, and the sense of smell is likely to fade sooner and more significantly than that of taste.

Finally, problems of general health can disrupt the sense of smell. Not uncommonly, a respiratory ailment, such as a cold, sinusitis or allergic congestion blocks the passage to the olfactory membranes with mucus and inflamed tissue. In some viral infections, especially influenza and viral hepatitis, congestion may be coupled with actual damage to the smell receptors. Most victims recover their sense of smell in time, but some, especially the elderly, suffer permanent loss or, perhaps even more troubling, a perversion of the sense of smell. Odors then have their normal potency but are experienced as unpleasant. Food in particular smells bad, and appetite and the pleasure of eating accordingly decline.

One victim, New Jersey pizza baker Rudy Coniglio, vividly recalled the very night in July 1969 when he was stricken. He was peeling a tomato, he said, and: "It smells rotten. It smells like garbage." Angrily, he telephoned his wholesaler. "He says I'm crazy—he don't handle rotten tomatoes." Coniglio went into his kitchen for fresh tomatoes, and the full extent of his affliction came home to him: "Did you ever when you're a kid burn a plastic comb? Everything in the kitchen smelled like that."

Because the chemical and nervous causes of the condition remain unexplained, clinical treatment is largely experimental. Certain medicines—vitamins and zinc, for example—have shown some effectiveness, but controlled trials have been too few to warrant full confidence in any one method.

A feast of tastes from sweet, salt, sour and bitter

As compared with its sister sense, smell, the sense of taste is simple. Scientists still argue about the number and identities of the basic smells; they generally agree upon four basic building blocks of taste—sweet, salt, sour and bitter—that combine to create all others. Human taste is relatively crude; on the average, it takes many more molecules to stimulate a taste sensation than it does to stimulate one of smell. And while the taste apparatus still contains some chemical mysteries, its parts and their locations are pretty well known.

The working parts of that apparatus are the taste buds, clustered in bumps, or papillae, on the surface of the tongue and scattered around the roof of the mouth. Each taste bud consists of about 50 cells; the mouth contains thousands of these sensory receptors.

A sensation of taste begins when a chemical dissolved in saliva flows around a papilla. The instant the solution makes contact with a receptor at extensions of the bud cells, the

TEMPERATURE AND TASTE
Most foods seem more flavorful when hot, but studies show that only the perception of sweetness intensifies as the temperature of the food increases, at least until it reaches body temperature—explaining why melted ice cream is so cloying. The reasons for the drops in intensities of other tastes remain a mystery.

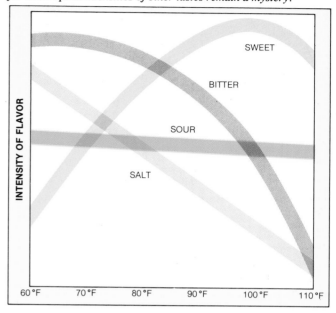

receptor undergoes a chemical change, and an electrical signal generated by the change goes to the brain.

The tongue varies widely in its sensitivity to the four primary tastes. It can detect the sweetness of sugar in a saliva solution at a concentration of one part in 200; table salt at one in 400; sourness, as in vinegar, at one in 15,000; and bitterness, as in quinine, at one in two million. This broad spectrum of sensitivity reflects the benefits and the dangers of foods. Generally, such naturally sweet foods as ripe fruits are energy producers, quickly digested and eaten in large quantities; sensitivity to them is comparatively dull precisely because the body uses large amounts of them. Salty foods help to maintain the balance of minerals in the body; the balance is critical, but delicate, and the taste buds respond sharply to small amounts of salt. Sour foods—particularly sour fruits that have not ripened to sweetness—are often inedible; high sensitivity to them represents a kind of warning. The highest sensitivity of all, and thus the most alert warning system, is for bitter chemicals, which often signal a natural poison.

Other factors modify or enhance tastes. To begin with, the tongue is the part of the body most sensitive to touch, temperature and pain. The texture of a food affects its flavor; children, particularly, often insist that rough or lumpy foods taste bad. Hot and cold foods, which trigger both taste and temperature receptors, inhibit the fullest sensation of such basic tastes as sweetness *(page 13);* professional tasters generally find their perceptions most acute when foods and beverages are taken at or near body temperature. For reasons not fully understood, some substances trigger heat and cold receptors when eaten at any temperature; thus, menthol stimulates a sensation of cold, and ginger or mustard one of heat. Finally, extreme temperatures and certain powerful spices that act as chemical irritants (such as chilies and other hot peppers) bring pain receptors into play, and their sensations, too, figure in the overall judgment of flavor.

Far more important than the tactile sensations of irritation and heat is the contribution of odor. Most of the impression thought of as taste actually arises by way of the sense of smell. The impacts of chocolate and vanilla, for example, lie primarily in their odors, and much of the experience of eating cheese is also based on aroma; a piece of Roquefort cheese eaten when the nasal passages are congested is hardly more flavorful than wax. Blocked nasal passages also make an apple and a raw potato taste almost exactly the same. Their textures and temperatures are identical, and their only true taste is one of slight sweetness; what is taken as a taste difference between them is in fact a difference of aroma.

Not only are flavors modified by other senses, but taste itself changes throughout life. For one thing, the cells within the taste buds constantly die and, to a greater or lesser extent, are constantly renewed. Bruised and battered by friction, by extremes of heat and cold, by the irritation of spices, they are regularly sloughed off and replaced by vigorous new ones about once every 10 days. Until recently it was generally assumed that the renewal rate slows drastically with age, and that older people are destined to lose all but a fraction of their taste sensitivity for this reason alone. New research has altered this view a little. Many factors can impair the sense of taste—disease, injury, smoking—and an older person has had much more time to be exposed to these things than a young one. Statistically, of course, there is more loss among

the elderly, and cell replacement slows in the tongue as it does everywhere else, but many healthy older people have a high degree of taste sensitivity.

Some researchers, however, point out that certain conditions linked to age probably do diminish tastes in older people. The sex hormone estrogen is essential to the generation of cells, and postmenopausal women, whose estrogen levels plummet, may be subject to an inevitable decline in taste sensitivity; at the age of 57, for example, Queen Victoria of England remarked mournfully that strawberries no longer tasted as sweet as they had in her childhood. A zinc deficiency, caused either by diet or by a malfunction in the body's absorption and storage of zinc, has also been blamed by some scientists for slow regeneration of taste buds.

A declining sense of taste can deprive its victim of more than the pleasures of the dining table. Many older people change their eating habits. Their diet may soon lack a healthful balance of essential nutrients. To make the most of a fading sense of taste, Dr. Maury Massler of Tufts University recently offered his patients four concrete suggestions:

• Choose foods that require chewing, and chew them thoroughly. Chewing increases salivation; salivation increases taste by dissolving more food chemicals and making them more available to the taste buds; and taste increases appetite. Thus, the best meals consist of small, bite-sized chunks of meat rather than ground-meat patties, fresh fruits with the skins on rather than mashed or cooked fruits, and such bite-resistant vegetables as carrots, green peppers and celery.

• When brushing the teeth, brush the tongue too, gently but thoroughly. Taste sensations will be improved by removal of heavy coatings, stale food particles and microorganisms.

• Stop smoking. Not only does smoking foul the mouth and diminish the taste for food, it also inhibits the sense of smell, which carries the main burden of sensory information in the enjoyment of food.

• Add reasonable amounts of aromatic seasonings and foods to enhance the flavors of a dish. Pepper, mustard, onion and fruit extracts are some of the more common ones.

In following the last precept, do not fall into the trap of adding excessive amounts of salt, sugar or harsh spices, for

Saving sight on an assembly line

In India some 5.5 million people, more than one in every 100, are totally blinded by cataracts, the clouding of the lens of the eye. No one can explain this very high rate—intense sunlight, malnutrition and poor hygiene may cause it—but the results are devastating. In an economy of scarcity, such as India's, blindness is life-threatening; unable to work and thus reduced to beggary, a blinded farmer can expect to live only a year or two.

To save the sight and lives of these people, the Indian government and Western philanthropies have set up temporary surgical camps in school buildings, public rooms, even marriage halls. At these roving clinics a surgeon may do as many as 300 cataract operations a day, slitting corneas and plucking out diseased lenses in a procedure that takes about two minutes. Nine out of 10 patients leave camp with their sight restored, and with a pair of free eyeglasses ground to a standard prescription. For an Indian farmer, custom-made glasses are not essential to a useful life. Said Dr. Harbans Singhe, a surgeon at one camp: "To be able to tell the difference between a cow and a goat is enough."

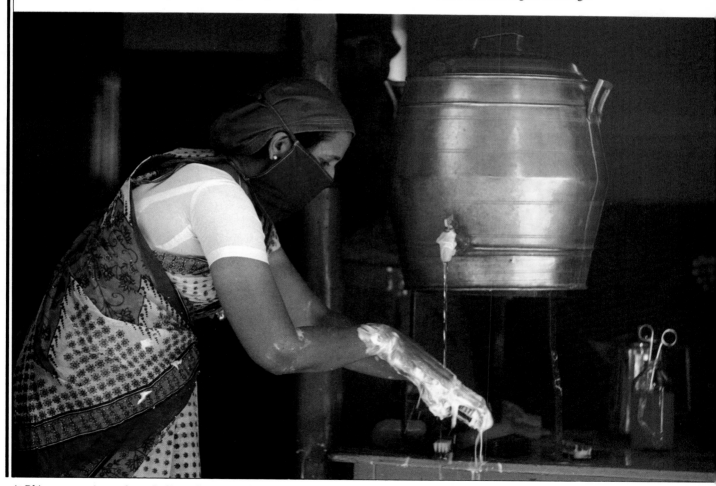

At Bhimavaram, in southeast India, a doctor scrubs her hands in preparation for a day of cataract surgery. The covered water jug is something of an amenity: At some eye camps surgeons scrub in open buckets filled from a communal village well.

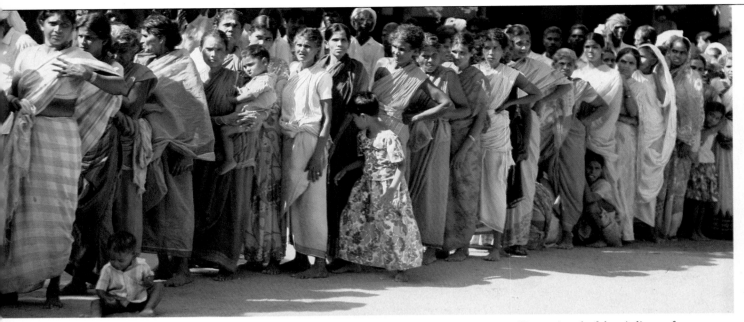

Women in colorful saris line up for diagnosis at an eye camp; male patients, dressed in white, form a separate line in the background. Relatives feed and care for all patients during their stay at the camp.

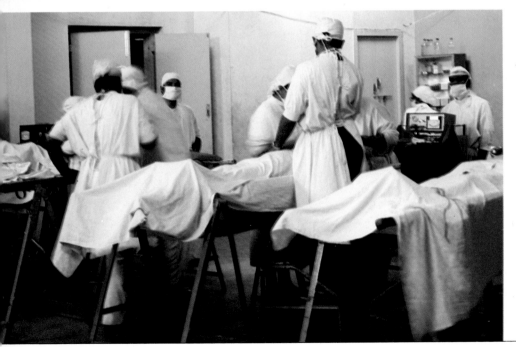

In a converted schoolroom, surgeons and assistants operate on three patients at a time. At the head of each operating table a special refrigerating unit chills the tip of a surgical probe used to extract a cataract-clouded lens; in less well-equipped camps, surgeons remove lenses just as quickly, though less neatly, with a pair of forceps.

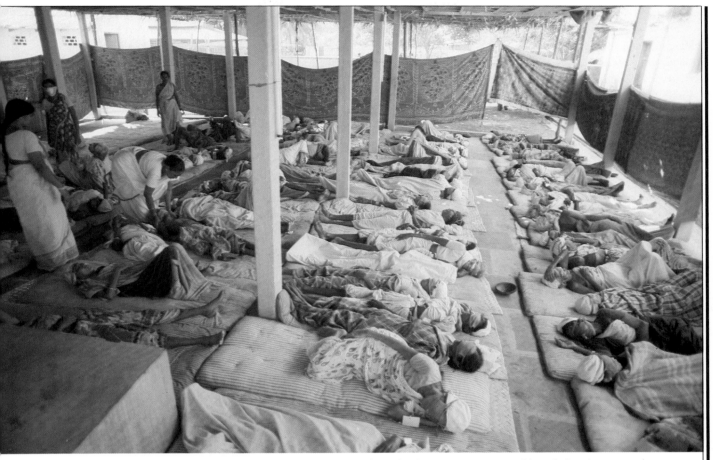

Convalescing patients are nursed by relatives in a women's recovery ward. Their stay in the ward lasts a week to 10 days; then a surgeon examines them, retrieves the eyeshades that were issued by the clinic, and sends them home.

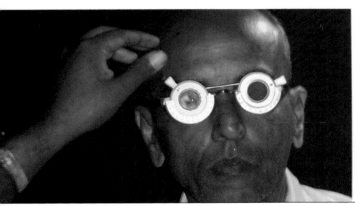

A recovered patient peers through a set of trial lenses as he is fitted for custom-made eyeglasses. The scene is unusual at the eye camps; the luxury of individual lens prescriptions is generally enjoyed only by the well to do.

each can have harmful effects of its own. One of the worst traps is overuse of the flavor-enhancing compound monosodium glutamate (MSG), sometimes adopted by people on low-sodium diets on the theory that it intensifies whatever salty taste is already present. MSG is itself a sodium compound in which the salt taste is weaker, grain for grain, than that of common table salt. Linda Bartoshuk of Yale University warned, ''If a person seasons food with MSG to the level of saltiness normally obtained with sodium chloride, the sodium content of that food will triple.''

Why people see better than animals

Although the primitive senses of touch, taste and smell remain surprisingly important to human beings, the two more advanced methods of perception, sight and hearing, are the ones most often used. The human eye, in particular, is remarkably versatile as a sensing device over a range of distances. Unlike most animal eyes, it can see distant objects—the thin mast of a ship 40 miles off at the horizon—as easily as the words of this book a foot away.

To achieve this versatility, a complex combination of bones, muscles, connective tissue, blood vessels and nerves is fitted into a small space. Bone forms the outermost structure, called the orbit—a rigid, protective socket formed by skull and facial bones. Within it, a lining of fatty tissue cushions blows and forms a friction-free surface in which the eyeball can rotate smoothly. (Permanent puffiness under the eyes is nothing more than fatty tissue that has slipped out of position.) Atop the orbit is the eyebrow, an awning against the noonday sun and a sweatband to catch dribbles from a steamy forehead.

At the opening of the socket, eyelids and lashes protect the eyes from dust, foreign objects and intense light. To close the lids, a muscle pulls the movable upper lid down against the lower; to open the eye, another muscle raises the upper lid. Within the lids, glands secrete tiny amounts of oil to slow tear evaporation and keep the eyelashes supple; the openings of these glands can be seen as a row of minute punctures just inside the lashes.

The innermost layer of the lids is a fold of moist, mucus-secreting membrane, called the conjunctiva, which laps over onto the eyeball itself. The conjunctiva is a kind of gasket, forming a tight, impenetrable seal between the front of the eyeball and the back. No object, however small or slippery (such as a contact lens, the most feared example), can slide or drift through this barrier to the back of the eye.

Nestled within the lids, just above the outer corner, are tear glands. At every wink, every closing of the eyelid, every tiny eye movement, the glands squeeze out a teardrop, which the lid spreads across the eyeball. Except for times when weeping overwhelms the system and the eye overflows with tears, the part of a tear that does not evaporate in the washing process drains out unnoticed through a pair of canals at the inner corner of the eyelids and flows into the nasal cavity.

Tears are primarily a protective device. Without them, the conjunctiva and the exposed surface of the eyeball would dry up, and friction would rub the eye raw. Tears also contain an antibacterial agent called lysozyme. First identified in 1922 by Alexander Fleming, the discoverer of penicillin, lysozyme is more powerful than carbolic acid, yet does not injure the fragile structures of the eye. The tear glands step up the production and concentration of lysozyme when the eye is threatened by infection. Dr. R. Linsy Farris of Columbia University notes, ''The more one tears, the more protected their eyes become against bacteria.''

As versatile as the eye's protective systems are its muscles. Six outside the eyeball, stretched between the eyeball and the orbit, move each eye in every direction and also coordinate its motions with that of the other eye. Both eyes can converge upon a nearby object or turn together. Normally, by a process called binocular vision, the two eyes fuse the separate images they see into a single picture.

For a distant object, binocular vision is relatively simple, since the images are virtually the same. But the eyes look at a nearby object from positions about three inches apart, and receive slightly disparate images. The brain not only fuses these separate pictures but makes their differences useful. It compares the two-dimensional view of the left eye with that of the right, and comes up with a three-dimensional, stereoscopic view that makes it possible to gauge the approximate size and shape of objects, to calculate distances and to move safely and efficiently in space.

Although the muscle actions that move and coordinate the eyes are usually involuntary, regulated without thought, they can be put under the conscious control of the brain. In some circumstances, making one eye look at one thing while the other looks at something else can be very useful. People who work with stereoscopic pictures—such as the military specialists who interpret aerial reconnaissance photographs—can train their eyes to focus separately, enabling the brain to fuse two images into one three-dimensional view. (A different trick is used by microscopists, who teach the brain to shut off the image transmitted by one eye; then they can keep that eye open, avoiding the strain of forcing it closed, while the other eye looks through the microscope.)

All of these coordinated movements and focusing operations are centered in the eyeball, a resilient, slightly egg-shaped body about one inch in diameter, filled to firmness with clear fluids and wrapped with membranes. It is designed essentially to receive and bend rays of light.

Bending light rays to converge in a sharp image on the back of the eyeball is the job of two structures at the front of the eye, the cornea and the lens. The cornea, a hard, clear pane, bulges outward from the sclera, a tough fibrous tissue that covers five sixths of the eyeball. The sclera is the opaque white of the eye—though it often looks faintly bluish in children, because it is still thin and translucent; and it may have a yellowish cast in the elderly from tiny deposits of fat.

The cornea is the eye's primary focusing element, about three times more powerful than the lens behind it. For most long-distance vision, the cornea does virtually all the focusing. The lens adds focusing power when an object is less than about 20 feet away and light rays must be bent beyond the powers of the fixed cornea. The lens, convex both front and back, is enclosed in a capsule-like sac, which in turn is suspended in a web of hairlike muscles and ligaments. For distant vision, these muscles relax and the ligaments pull the lens into a shape that is only slightly convex; when closer vision is called for, muscles automatically contract, pulling the ligaments so that the lens thickens and bulges. This gives

the lens-cornea combination enough refractive (or light-bending) power to focus upon objects only inches away.

Between the cornea and the lens is the iris, a doughnut-shaped sheet of pigmented muscle directly behind the cornea. The hole in the doughnut is the pupil, which serves the same purpose as the lens opening of a camera; it is adjusted by the iris to control the amount of light passing through the lens. When the light level drops, the iris muscle relaxes, the sides of the iris narrow and the pupil opening enlarges to admit more light. In bright light the process is reversed; less light strikes the back of the eye. A fully enlarged pupil is about 16 times the area of one fully constricted.

The iris gives the eye its color. Irises come in many shades—blue, gray, green, brown and almost everything in between (appropriately, the word iris stems from the Greek word for rainbow). Yet only one pigment, melanin, supplies all shades, the color depending on its concentration; the more dense the melanin, the browner the iris. Paradoxically, blue-eyed people have almost no pigment at all: The front of the iris admits all colors of light; red and green light is absorbed at the back of the iris, while blue light is bounced outward by fibers in the top layer, creating the appearance of blue.

The innermost membrane of the eyeball is the retina, a gossamer-fine membrane that contains the specialized sensors of vision. These nerve cells respond to the energy in light rays, converting them into an electrical code. The coded message passes through bundles of nerve fibers; the bundles merge in a main trunk line, the optic nerve; and the nerve runs through the back of the eye socket and on to the brain.

The eye contains two kinds of sensing cells, both named for their shapes. Cones are adapted to a world of bright light and color, rods to one of dimness and shadows. Six million plump cones—about a million of them concentrated in the fovea, a pinhead-sized area at the center of the retina, and in a slightly larger surrounding area called the macula—record brightness and color. Each cone contains one of three pigments, sensitive to one of three colors: blue, green or red. Stimulated in an almost infinite variety of numbers and combinations, the cones can distinguish more than 150 hues.

In dim light the cones are no longer sensitive to stimula-

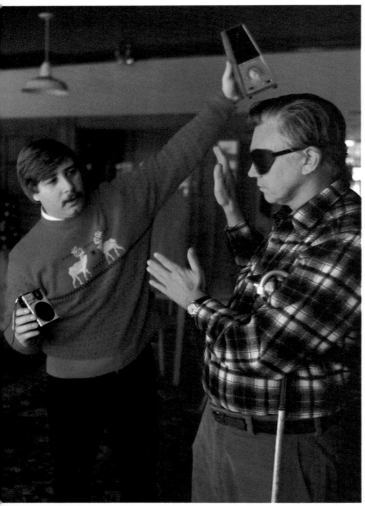

Learning to orient himself with sound, recently blinded Thomas Cole gestures toward a radio and metronome held by Paul Arathuzik, a teacher at the Carroll Center for the Blind in Newton, Massachusetts. Cole uses the two sound sources as reference points—imagining them as corners of a triangle—and compares their direction and distance to get a fix on his own position.

tion. Then the retina's 123 million slender rods take over, recording only black, white and shades of gray. The rods are extremely sensitive to light energy and to movement; they warn the brain immediately of hazards out of the corner of the eye. Rods are absent in the fovea, relatively sparse in the macula, and predominant in the remainder of the retina, where they provide protective peripheral vision. Like the cones, rods respond to light by means of a pigment—in their case, a pigment called rhodopsin.

Both rods and cones transform the energy of light into electrical impulses through chemical changes in their pigment molecules. Some of the details of the process, particularly in the cones, are not fully understood, but what is known about the transformation of rhodopsin in the rods probably applies to both types of sensors. A rod contains some 10 million rhodopsin molecules, stacked like beads to the surface of the retina. When light strikes the outermost molecule, it breaks down into two nonpigment molecules, retinene and scotopsin. This chemical change, comparable to the change in which light bleaches the pigments of a fabric, sets off the electrical impulses that pass through the optic nerve. Every day countless numbers of pigment molecules are destroyed at the top of a rod and countless others are synthesized at the bottom.

The eye's greatest acuity occurs within the fovea, partly because cones are jammed together there, but also because each cone has its own transmission line to the brain. In the rest of the retina, rods and cones share nerve fibers, and the mixed linkages produce messages to the brain that are less well defined, less specific, coarser.

The part of the optic nerve that lies within an eye socket is about an inch long; this length allows for all the turning the eye can do. Less than half an inch beyond the socket, the trunk line meets the optic nerve of the other eye. Here, in one of the most intricate anatomical arrangements in the human body, about half of the fibers from each eye's optic nerve cross over to join the remaining fibers of the opposite nerve. The shunted fibers are not selected at random; they are the fibers linked to receptors on the half of each retina closest to the nose. Ultimately, the right optic trunk line sends the brain messages about the left side of the field of vision; the left trunk line delivers only the signals from the right side of the field. In ways not yet fully understood, the brain uses this formidably complex routing system to make the exchanges of information that are essential to binocular vision.

With so much delicate machinery operating in the eyeball and along the pathways of vision, it is something of a miracle that human eyes are not constantly troubled by disorders. In fact, during a lifetime of constant use, most people experience only occasional eye irritation or minor infection and some degree of focusing error, both easily correctible. More serious threats to sight, however, are on the rise; these include such diseases as cataracts, glaucoma and retinal disorders. In the main, the diseases are treatable if attended to promptly, either with medication or by modern surgery. The greatest danger lies in ignoring them until the damage they cause is beyond repair.

Hearing: the sense that is always turned on

Although the eye is wonderfully versatile in its parts and functions, the ear is even more so. To begin with, an ear houses not one sense, but two. A set of ear sensors provides the brain with raw material for the sense of hearing; another serves as a kind of automatic pilot for the body, monitoring posture, balance and movement.

Hearing is the more important of these two senses, because sound is so pervasive and vital to human beings. Sounds move through darkness as well as through light, and human ears have no convenient covers, comparable to eyelids, for shutting them out. What is more, sound moves easily around small barriers; ears can hear around a corner. Most important of all, human beings generate their own sounds, including the varied, subtle sounds of language that make human beings peculiarly human.

All sound consists of waves of pressure, traveling through a medium—generally, for human beings, the medium of air. The waves are produced by mechanical vibration—the vibration of vocal cords, of a violin string, of one car fender striking another, or indeed of any other object rapidly moving back and forth. The movement sends forth alternate vol-

leys of pressure and rarefaction that move through the air at hundreds of miles per hour. The degree of compression and rarefaction determines the sound intensity, perceived as the loudness of a sound, from a whisper to a roar. The rate at which alternations occur determines its frequency, perceived as the pitch of the sound, from the lowest rumble to the highest squeak.

To convert the intensity and frequency of pressure alternations into the intelligible distinctions of loudness and pitch, the hearing mechanism includes a strange variety of parts, some little more than flaps of skin, others extremely intricate. An outer ear scoops in sound waves, a middle ear transmits and concentrates them in a space no bigger than a pea, and an inner ear converts them into an electrical code for the brain to interpret.

The outer ear gathers sound by means of an external flap and an auditory canal. The flap, composed mostly of cartilage enveloped by a thin layer of skin, lies like a crumpled ear trumpet alongside the head. A vestigial version of the more prominent, movable ear of other animals, it not only helps direct sound waves into the ear but also provides some protection to the more fragile chambers within the head.

The auditory canal is a narrowing channel about an inch long that ends at the eardrum, or tympanum, where the middle ear begins. Along the outer third of its length, the canal is lined with glands that secrete a protective ear wax, which coats its surface; some studies indicate that the taste and odor of the wax is repellent to intruding insects. The eardrum itself is a delicate, easily punctured membrane, stretched taut as a drumhead and equally responsive to sound waves. Except when injured, it forms an effective barrier against germs, dust and water.

Behind the eardrum lies the middle ear, an air-filled cavity about $1/3$ inch wide and $1/6$ inch deep, protected by some of the hardest bones in the human body. The cavity is lined with a mucous membrane, which also runs along the walls of a slender channel, the Eustachian tube, to the larger cavity and mucous membrane of the nose and throat. The tube has an important function: It balances air pressure on the inner and outer sides of the eardrum. But it is by this route that colds

The adhesive patch behind this man's ear contains scopolamine, a drug that is absorbed into the bloodstream through the skin to prevent motion sickness. Its effect lasts as long as three days, eliminating the need for frequent pill-taking. Scopolamine apparently turns off those nerves of the balance organ in the inner ear that connect with the nausea center in the brain.

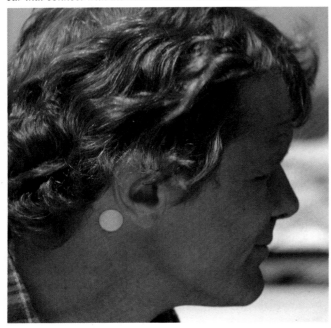

and other respiratory infections occasionally invade the ear.

In the middle ear, between the eardrum and the inner wall of the cavity, three tiny bones form a transmission bridge for sound. The vibrating eardrum sets the first of them, the hammer, in motion; the hammer relays the vibration to a smaller bone, the anvil; and the anvil passes the vibration on to the third and smallest bone, the stirrup, which sits in an opening called the oval window—the entrance to the inner ear.

Sound waves do not as a rule carry much energy. When they strike the solid surface of the eardrum, most of the energy they do have bounces back and is lost to hearing. But the bones of the middle ear take full advantage of the energy that does get through—indeed, they must do so, to overcome what engineers would call an "impedance mismatch" between the outer and inner ears. The outer ear is filled with air, a highly compressible gas; the inner ear, with a nearly incompressible fluid. If the outer ear were in direct contact with the inner, so that the eardrum lay directly between a compressible gas and an incompressible fluid, sound waves would never reach the inner ear; instead, they would all bounce back from the rigid drum into the compliant air.

The middle-ear bones bridge the gap—in engineering language, they match impedances—by transmitting and increasing the force of eardrum movement through a solid medium. Part of the increase comes from a mechanical advantage—the hammer and anvil bones operate as levers—but the greater part is effected by concentrating the force on ever-smaller areas. As it passes the vibration of the drum along, the hammer concentrates the pressure on the smaller anvil, and the anvil on the still smaller stirrup. When the mechanical thrust reaches the oval window, only $1/20$ the area of the eardrum, its pressure per square inch has been increased as much as 50 times.

With the help of this increase, the ear can sense a movement of as little as two billionths of an inch in the eardrum. Yet noises 100 trillion times louder than the softest audible sound are handled safely. When very loud noises strike, muscles automatically tighten the drum, reduce the vibration of the hammer and ease the stirrup away from the oval window.

Beyond the oval window lie the sensors for hearing and balance. The organs involved in hearing are fitted into a spiraling bony structure called the cochlea, one of the most extraordinary examples of miniaturization in the human body. No bigger than the tip of the little finger, the cochlea is capable of exquisite sensitivity and herculean labor.

The cochlea is a tube divided into three ducts, coiled two and a half times around itself, and filled with fluids. The top and bottom ducts are rigid, bony canals; wedged between them is the flexible cochlear duct, containing three key components of reception—the basilar and tectorial membranes, and the organ of Corti.

Sound enters the inner ear when the stirrup moves in and out of the oval window and sets the fluid at the entrance of the cochlea into vibration. Now transformed into vibrations in liquid, a sound wave passes almost instantaneously along the upper duct, round the bend at the coiled apex of the cochlea, and back through the bottom duct to the round window, a membrane just below the oval window, where the vibrations are dissipated. During their passage through the bottom duct, the traveling waves undulate the basilar membrane, the lower wall of the cochlear duct. This delicate membrane is narrow and stiff at the end nearest the oval window, but increasingly wide, loose and supple as it proceeds through the cochlea's spiral; by contrast, the tectorial membrane, which forms the upper wall of the duct, is stiff throughout its length. As pressure waves roll over the basilar membrane, sounds are separated out according to their frequency: High frequencies produce the greatest bulges at the near end, where the membrane is taut; low tones have most effect at the far end, where the membrane is slack.

Lying alongside the membrane and following its every move is the organ of Corti, consisting of countless hairlike receptors that respond to vibration whenever they are bent. As waves travel along the basilar membrane, causing one point or another to undulate, the receptors at each point bend against the stiff overlying tectorial membrane—and this shearing action produces electrical charges at the base of the receptors. The stimulus to hearing began as an airborne sound wave in the outer ear. It became a vibration of solid bones in the middle ear, and a hydraulic wave in the fluids of the inner ear. Now it is transformed at last into an electrical code. The electrical impulses flow along some 30,000 fibers that make up the auditory nerve, which runs to the brain.

This complex process of reception and coding goes on not once, but twice, for every sound—because hearing takes place in both the left and right ears. Two-eared, or binaural, hearing enhances the ability to hear: A process called binaural summation makes hearing almost twice as sensitive with two ears as with one. More important, the use of two ears enables a hearer to locate the source of a sound. Normally, a sound is perceived by the ears as two separate and subtly different sounds: The ear nearer to the source of sound hears it a fraction of a second sooner, and it hears a slightly louder sound because the head partially blocks the pathway to the far ear. By analyzing the minuscule differences of loudness and arrival time, the brain can generally tell where the sound is coming from.

The brain also decodes a second set of messages from the inner ear—signals having to do with balance and movement.

The organ for these sensations consists of three hollow fluid-filled loops called the semicircular canals. Each loop lies in a different plane, like walls and floor at the corner of a room—two loops vertical at right angles and one approximately horizontal. Each contains a free-swinging flap covered with sensory hairs that respond to bending in much the same way as the receptors of the organ of Corti. When the head moves, fluid in one or another loop surges against the flap and bends the hairs, sending an electrical signal to the part of the brain that controls the skeletal muscles. If necessary, the muscles involved are mobilized—a contraction here, a relaxation there—and balance is restored.

Overstimulation of the semicircular canals can overwhelm the brain's ability to unscramble the messages; the child riding a merry-go-round gets dizzy, and the sailor tossed by a choppy sea gets seasick. Why upsetting the balance organ should upset the stomach is a mystery. It does so in many animals—including, oddly, some fishes.

Some experts attribute seasickness to crossed wires in the brain, a happenstance of evolution that introduced seasickness as a side effect of a valuable protection against poisoning. Poisons that affect the nervous system, such as lead, affect vision or muscular coordination, which also are involved in the sense of balance. Such poisons are so dangerous that the body must react instantly by vomiting. As this protective response evolved, any derangement of balance, whether caused by poison or by something as harmless as the pitching of a boat, came to be associated by the brain with a threat to the nervous system—a threat to be answered with nausea.

Seasickness is seldom more than a temporary discomfort—and now can be prevented with reliable medicines (opposite). But balance, like the other senses, is prey to more serious attack, such as the chronic disorder called Ménière's disease, which must often be treated by advanced surgical procedures (page 122). The development of such therapies is vital to health. All of the senses, including the ones that people rarely worry about, are important to well-being. They are worth protecting, and more than is generally realized can be done to maintain their marvelous ability to tell the brain what is out there in the surrounding world. ✱

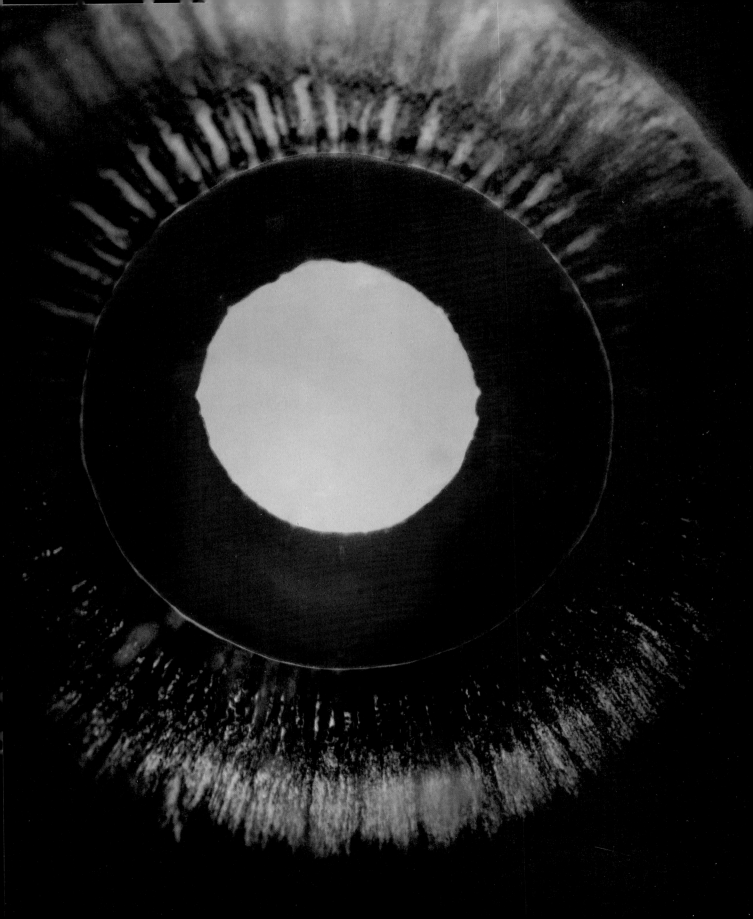

The delicate instruments of perception

Eagles see details farther off than humans, dogs hear fainter sounds, and salmon discern more delicate tastes—but human beings surpass all animals with a range of sharp senses. Delicate organs, near the surface of the human body, respond to an array of outside forces—light, sound, heat, chemical actions and many kinds of movement and pressure—then convert these forces into nerve signals that tell the brain what is going on around the body.

Scientists have now identified several parts of the brain that specialize in decoding signals from each sense *(below)*. The visual center, for example, is a relatively flat area at the back of the brain that receives eye signals in reverse—objects at the right side of the view register in the left side of the visual center, and vice versa. But then these signals go to other parts of the brain, where they are reversed again and correlated with signals from other senses. In the human brain a visual map also records sound signals because the ears as well as the eyes locate objects. (In the brain of certain pythons, a similar center responds not only to eye and ear nerves but to signals from 13 pairs of eyelike "pits" that sense heat and thus help the snake locate its prey.)

Information comes to the brain from nerves that end in clusters of receptors, as incredibly small as they are numerous. Leonardo da Vinci expressed his puzzlement at the power of the human eye, "Who would believe that so small a space could contain the images of all the universe?" Today, physiologists can explain: 130 million microscopic receptors, called rods and cones, cover the back of the eye and connect to the optic nerve.

The senses of hearing and sight require complex accessories that enable the receptors to work: in the ear, a chain of bones, tubes and membranes; in the eye, optical focusing elements, adjustable parts and muscles. But the more primitive senses of touch, taste and smell, sampling a world of textures, flavors and fragrances directly with nerve endings, need no such middlemen.

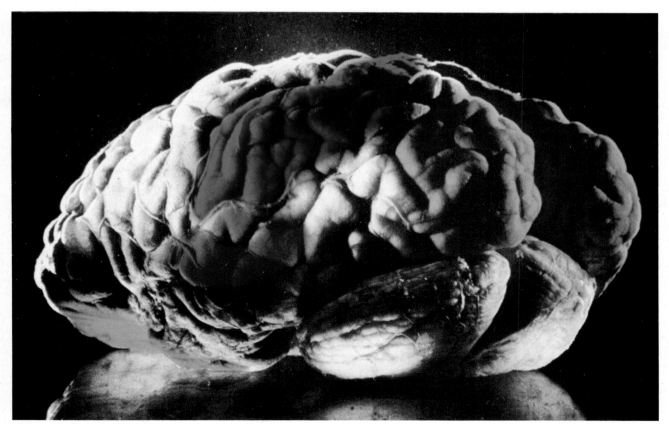

PHOTOGRAPHS BY LENNART NILSSON

From within an eye removed in an autopsy, blue sky is seen through the pupil, the opening in the iris. The striations around the iris are ligaments to hold and adjust the lens.

The areas of the brain that receive and relay sense signals are indicated approximately by the colors in this photograph: The yellow region controls sight, the reddish area touch. The small blue spot identifies a region, deep inside the brain, that registers tastes; nearby is hearing (orange). The seat of smell (green) lies at the underside of the brain, over the nose.

Diverse sensors in the skin

Touch is not one sense, but a broad class of discrete feelings—pain, cold, vibration and pressure, among many others. To distinguish them, human skin is provided with not one kind of sensor, but many. Each is a specialized receptor designed to report one kind of stimulus, although it may be activated by other stimuli if they are very strong: Powerful pressure, for example, can set off a perception of cold.

The receptors are quite dissimilar in size, shape and cell structure *(right)*, and they are unevenly distributed. Some inhabit only hair-covered skin, others only hairless skin. Tactile body parts such as fingertips contain more than the usual share of touch receptors, providing heightened sensitivity there. And several types of receptors have yet to be discovered: The search goes on for the receptor that feels heat, but the one that senses cold has already been identified.

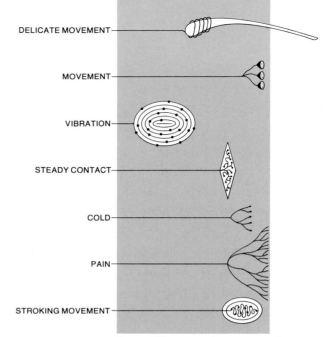

Seven different touch receptors, shown above at the ends of their connecting nerves, have been positively identified. They are sketched to scale and at their relative depths below the skin surface.

DELICATE MOVEMENT
Entwined around a hair root, this receptor fires at the slightest deflection of the hair.
MOVEMENT
Generally grouped under a dome of skin, this cluster reacts to any moving touch that also presses the skin down.
VIBRATION
The large vibration receptor responds only to momentary contact or vibration.
STEADY CONTACT
These spread-out nerve endings are activated whenever the skin is pushed.
COLD
A small and bulblike terminal reacts when the temperature of the skin surface drops by as little as .2° F.
PAIN
Spreading over a larger area than any of the others do, this receptor ignores minor contacts but is excited by stimuli that may cause damage to tissue.
STROKING MOVEMENT
An oval disk, also shown in the photograph at right, detects a touch moving across hairless skin.

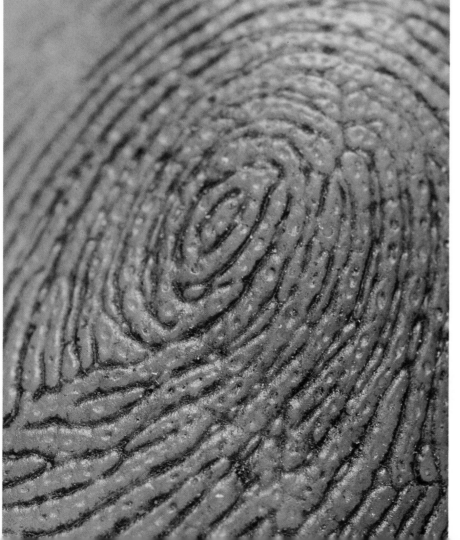

Beneath the whorl of this fingertip lies one of the body's most sensitive regions, skin containing 35,000 to 50,000 nerve endings per square inch.

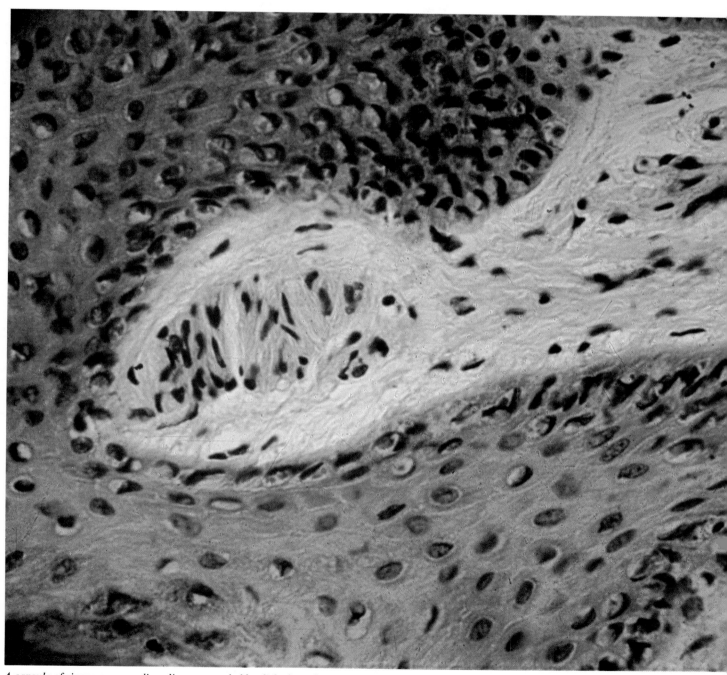

A capsule of zigzag nerve endings lies surrounded by disk-shaped cells of the skin surface, ready to fire off nerve impulses if squeezed by a moving touch on the hairless area it serves. This receptor, sketched at bottom in the illustration on the opposite page, is called a Meissner's corpuscle, after the 19th Century anatomist-physiologist who discovered it.

The supersensitive nose

Smell, a sense whose evolutionary history extends back perhaps 500 million years, is provided in human beings by a membrane about the size of a small olive pit, located in the nasal passage. This so-called olfactory epithelium is covered with millions of hair-shaped projections, the odor-sensitive cilia, so small that they can be seen only with an electron microscope. The hairs make up the sensing end of the receptor cells—as many as 20 hairs to a cell—which respond to odor by sending a nerve signal to the brain. Next to each receptor cell are supporting cells, which secrete mucus that is believed to assist in catching odors.

The hairs react chemically to molecules in the air passing through the nose. A single molecule of some substances is enough to initiate the response, setting off a cascade of other chemical reactions, each more powerful than the last, in the receptor cell. Eventually the energy released is sufficient to fire the cell and signal the brain.

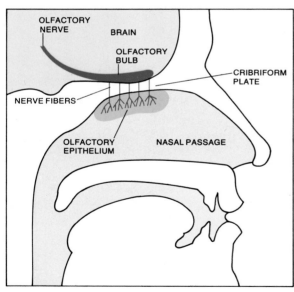

WHERE THE OLFACTORY ORGANS ARE
The olfactory epithelium, the smell-sensing membrane of the nose, is located at the ceiling of the nasal passage. From its receptor cells, nerve fibers pass through tiny holes in the cribriform plate, the bony floor under the front of the brain. The fibers converge at the olfactory bulb and unite into a large nerve that proceeds to the brain.

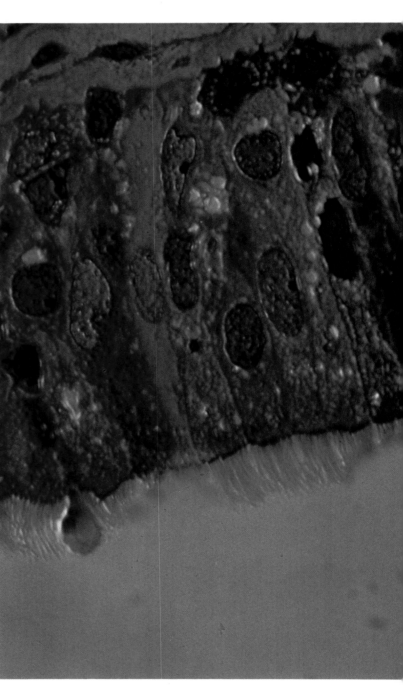

In this magnified cross section of olfactory epithelium, stained pink for clarity, odor-sensitive cilia form a fringe along the lower edge. The cilia project from column-shaped receptor cells; adjacent supporting cells secrete mucus.

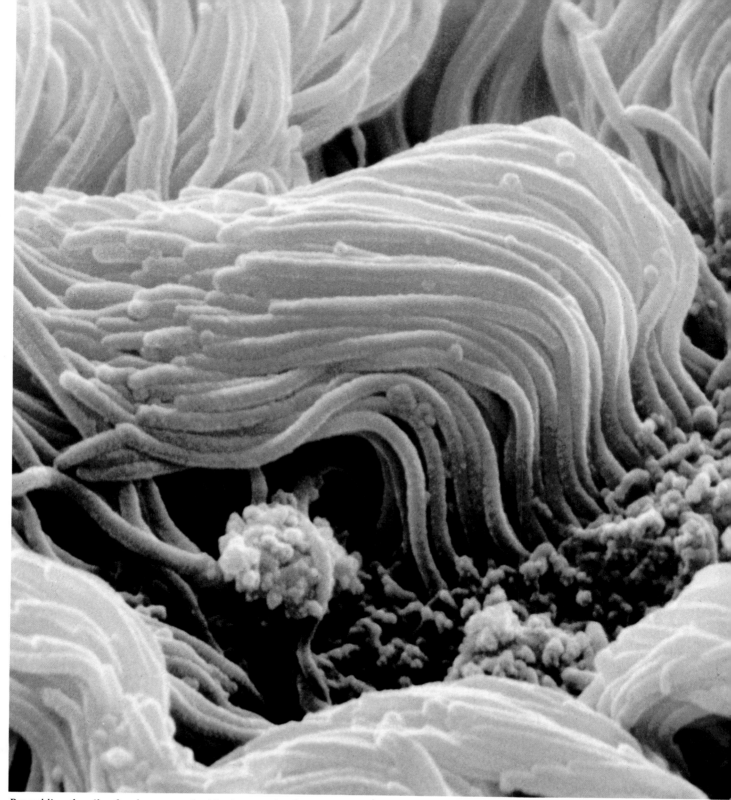

Resembling the pile of a shag carpet in this photograph taken with an electron microscope, cilia cells are bathed by a flow of mucus secretions. The mucus serves the cilia in two ways: It traps odor molecules and delivers nutrients.

Buds to savor tastes

Tastes and smells are often hard to distinguish, because what the brain perceives when something is eaten may be simply flavor—a combination of the two senses. Yet the signals sent to the brain have separate origins. Taste arises in buds embedded in the tongue, the roof of the mouth and, to a lesser extent, the throat *(right)*.

These buds are housed inside bumps of tissue known as papillae. Like the smell receptors of the olfactory epithelium, the taste buds have hairs that are chemically sensitive, but they react only to substances dissolved in saliva. All taste buds respond at least slightly to all of the four basic tastes— sour, sweet, salt and bitter—but as the drawings at right indicate, some are more sensitive to certain tastes than to others. Little taste is picked up by the center of the tongue, where there are few buds of any kind; the greatest concentration of receptors is at the back of the tongue.

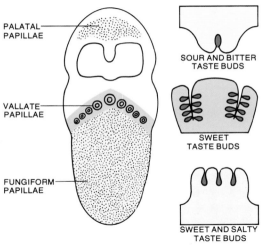

WHERE THE TASTE BUDS ARE
Taste buds, located in three parts of the mouth (sketched at left above as seen looking into a mouth agape), are shown in red inside bumps called papillae (right, above). From the tip of the tongue upward, in the drawing, are taste buds most sensitive to: sweet and salty, sweet, and sour and bitter tastes.

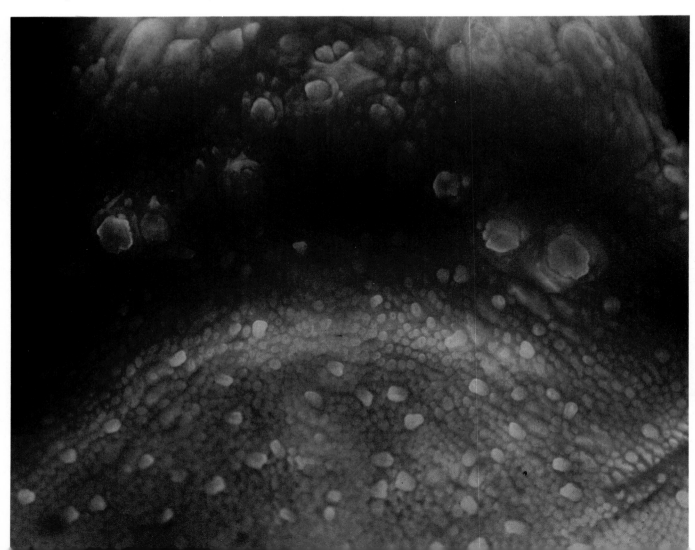

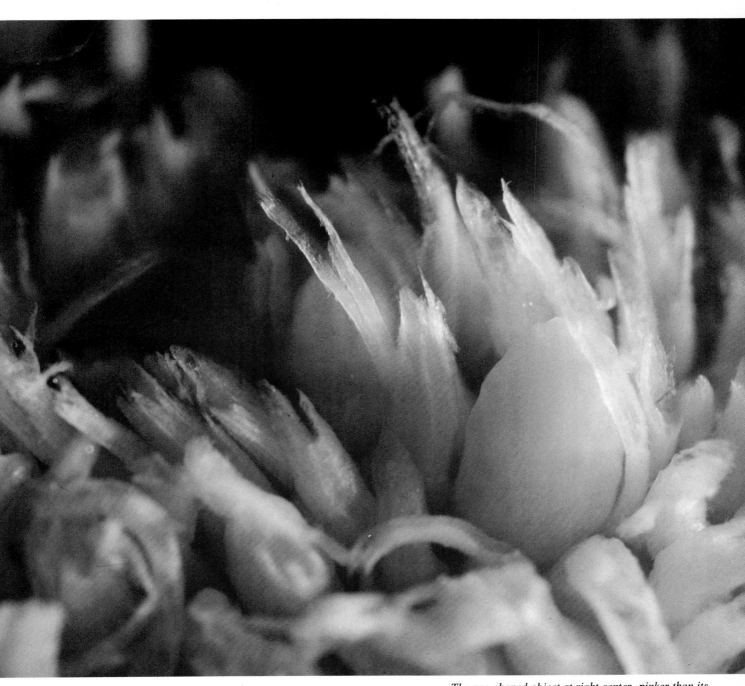

Arrayed near the back of the tongue, the large, rounded bumps seen at left are vallate papillae, housing sweet-loving taste buds. The smaller flecks are fungiform papillae, dotting the tongue to its tip with buds for sweetness and saltiness.

The egg-shaped object at right center, pinker than its surroundings, is a fungiform papilla, containing as many as eight taste buds. Around it is a thicket of hairlike filiform papillae, stiff projections that help move food but do not taste it.

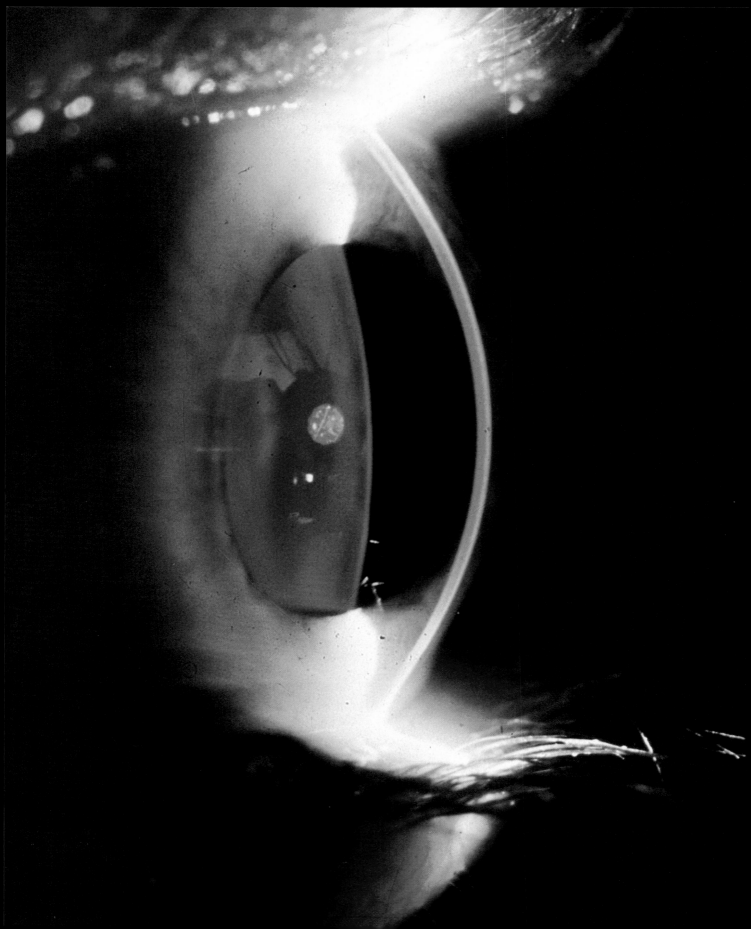

A complex eye for superior sight

Superior sight is a relatively recent evolutionary development—a heritage of life in the trees—that humans share mainly with a few other mammals and with birds. In addition to light-sensitive nerve endings, sharp vision requires an eyelid and iris to limit the incoming light, a cornea and lens to focus an image, muscles to move and adjust the parts, and clear fluids to hold everything in position.

The image thus formed registers on the retina, a thin layer of receptors spread over the curved back wall of the eye. There are two types of receptors, named for their shapes: more than 120 million rods, which pick up the image fuzzily in gray and white but give a broad picture and respond to dim light; and 6 million cones, concentrated in the center, or macula, which require bright light but distinguish colors and perceive fine details.

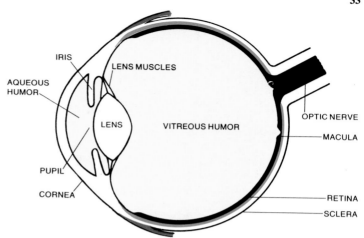

INSIDE THE EYE
The white sclera encases the eyeball except at the cornea, where light enters to pass through the iris pupil opening and lens, both adjusted by muscles. Supporting them is fluid, the aqueous humor. Vitreous humor helps secure the retina, whose light-detecting cells communicate with the brain via the optic nerve.

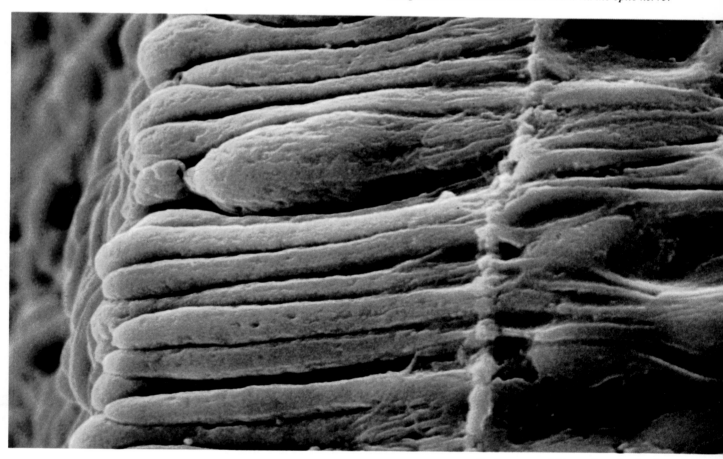

Revealed in profile behind the curve of the cornea (right), an eye lens—although actually colorless—appears as a blue oval ringed by a white iris. Both colors, like the white dot on the lens, are photographic distortions created by a strong spotlight.

In the center of this section of retina is a thick cone, a receptor sensitive to color and detail. Around it are rods; about 20 times more numerous than cones in the retina, they are responsible for peripheral vision and seeing in dim light.

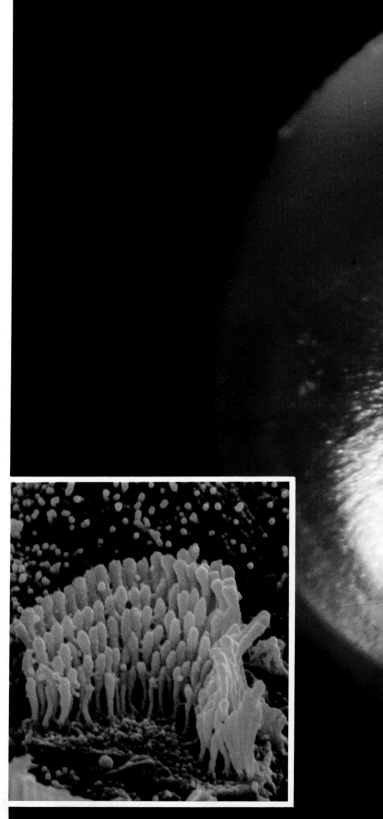

The intricate pathway of sound

The ear is a remarkable collection of living machinery, partly because it houses organs for both hearing and balance, but also because hearing requires a sequence of steps, each very delicate. Sounds—rhythmic movements of air molecules—are picked up by the external ear, which funnels them in to vibrate the eardrum membrane. The drum moves three linked bones, two named for their functions, hammer and anvil, the third for its shape, stirrup. The stirrup transmits its motion through the oval window, to move the fluid inside the cochlea, a chamber containing delicate hairs. These are the sound receptors; the fluid motion makes them signal the brain.

The balance organ—which evolved along with the hearing devices from a pressure sensor in fishes—also contains hairs that sense fluid motion. But these motions are caused by gravity when the head moves.

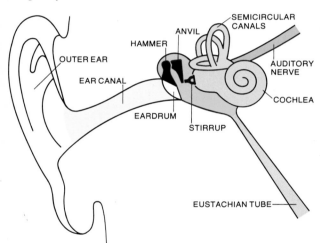

INSIDE THE EAR
The outer ear brings sound to the eardrum, attached to the three moving bones of the middle ear. They pass vibrations into the fluid-filled cochlea of the inner ear and its receptor cells (inset, right). Two other vital parts of the ear conduct no sound: The semicircular canals are the balance organ; the Eustachian tube is a vent that equalizes air pressure on both sides of the eardrum.

The parts of the middle ear, photographed from inside a cadaver ear looking out, are, left to right: the eardrum, bright because of light entering from outside, and the delicate bones that are triggered by the eardrum's vibrations. The hammer, attached to the eardrum, loosely touches the anvil (front-to-back in center). The anvil touches the stirrup, which is connected to the cochlea of the inner ear, where the sound-sensing cells are located (inset).

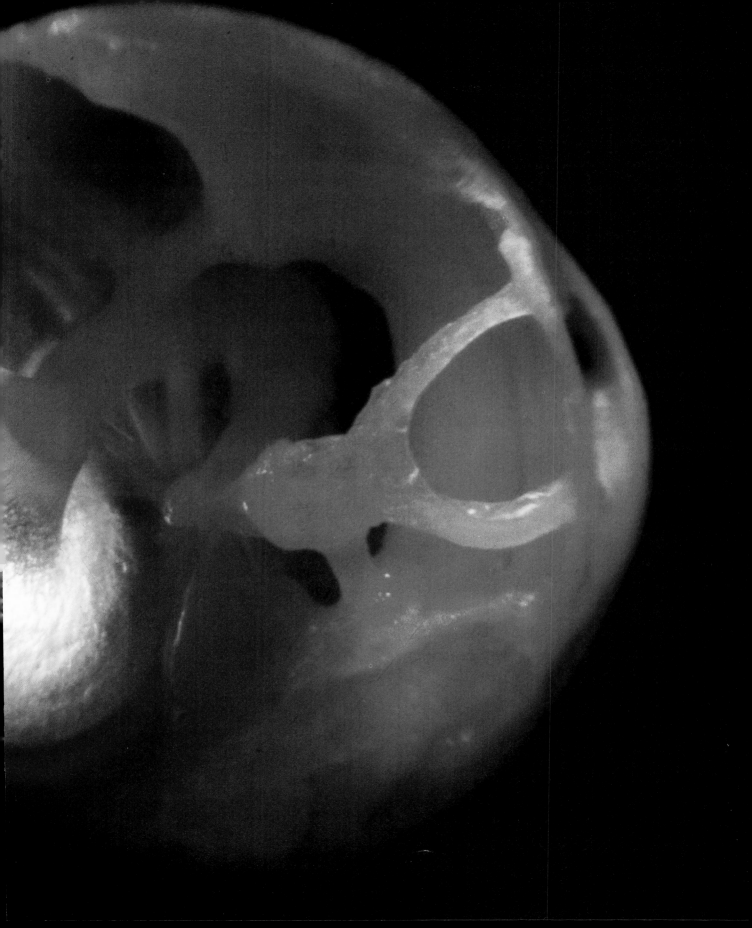

How to save your hearing

In a letter written many years ago, Helen Keller, who had been blind and deaf since the age of two, told a friend which handicap had proved more onerous. "Deafness is a much worse misfortune," she said, "for it means the loss of the most vital stimulus—the sound of the voice that brings language, sets thought astir, and keeps us in the intellectual company of man."

Because the ability to hear determines, in large measure, an individual's ability to communicate with others, much else rides on it. Hearing is critical to success in school and on the job, to feeling self-confident and accepted—in short, to winning and holding a place in human society. Such a vital sense demands protection, and safeguarding it can be easy and effective.

Although some hearing inexorably disappears as the years pass, more can be preserved than is generally realized. The most common impediment to good hearing is nothing but excess wax in the outer-ear canal—an obstruction that can usually be removed at home. More insidious thieves of hearing are noise and infection, either of which, if persistent, can cause permanent harm. Yet noise damage can be avoided by commonsense measures, such as the use of inexpensive earplugs by those operating power tools. And the cumulative deterioration brought on by repeated infection can be prevented by prompt care of earaches, for modern antibiotics usually eliminate infections before they can hurt hearing. Even when prevention fails and hearing diminishes, as it generally does with age, electronic aids or surgery *(Chapter 5)* often can restore at least some of what has been lost.

The first step in maintaining good hearing is keeping the passageways into the ears open, free of obstruction. Some people, however, go too far and wage war on dirt in the canal—or rather, on what they regard as dirt. They persist in poking deep into their ears—with fingers, cotton swabs or even hairpins or pencils—sometimes irritating the ear canal, puncturing the eardrum or, likeliest of all, driving the obstruction deeper into the ear to form a hard, immovable plug.

"Never put anything smaller than your elbow in your ear," doctors like to tell their patients, with a certain wry solemnity. The admonition against overzealous ear cleaning applies whether the object being cleaned out is a foreign intruder, such as water or an insect, or that native of the canal, wax. The battle against wax, in particular, often amounts to overkill. Ear wax is a normal, natural and desirable secretion of glands lining the outer ear. It moisturizes and protects the ears in much the same manner that tears nurse the surface of the eyes and mucus the nasal passages. What is more, ear wax plays a role in preventing infection, principally by trapping bacteria that otherwise could work deeper into the ear and, finding a more hospitable environment there, cause trouble.

For most people, most of the time, the ear does an admirable job of keeping itself clean. The wax, after gradually collecting dust, microscopic organisms and sloughed-off skin cells, dries and crumbles into tiny pellets. No longer sticky and able to cling to the ear canal, the pellets are shaken

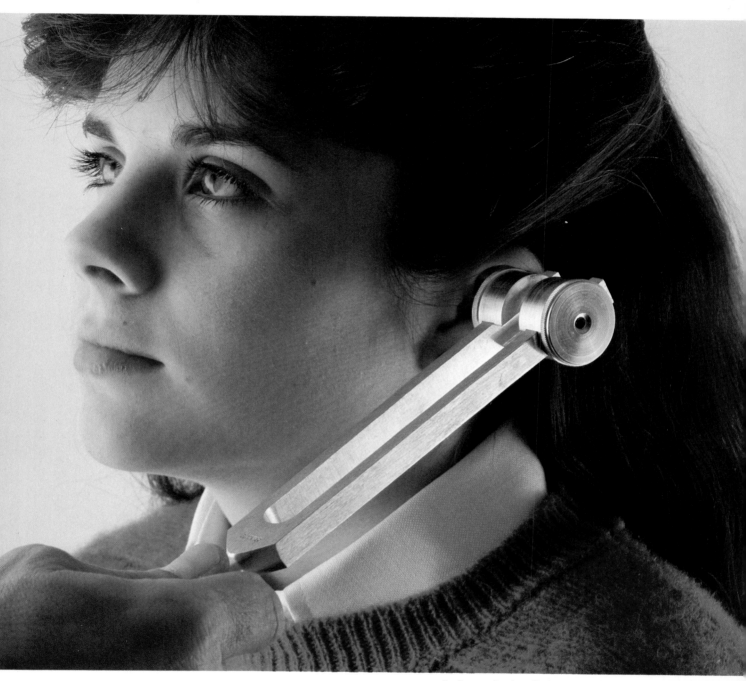

In the standard preliminary test of hearing, a physician vibrates a tuning fork outside a patient's ear to check normal perception of sound through the air. He also touches the fork to her skull behind her ear, transmitting sound via bone. If all is well, the tone will take twice as long to fade away through air as through bone, a less efficient transmission medium.

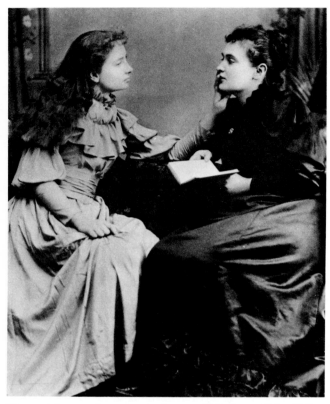

The most famous victor over deafness and blindness, Helen Keller, communicates by touch with her teacher Anne Sullivan in this 1890s photograph. Stricken in infancy, she painfully learned to speak, read Braille and write with a typewriter. In books and lectures, she inspired handicapped people everywhere with accounts of her liberation from darkness and silence.

loose by movement and migrate outward, to be washed away in the next bath. The best method for keeping the ears clear of wax, then, is to do nothing: Let the ears clean themselves, with an assist from bath water.

Occasionally the ears fail to do their own job of housecleaning. Some people produce wax faster than the ear can get rid of it. In others, long ear hairs trap the wax, or an unusually curved or narrow ear canal prevents it from falling out. Muffled hearing is a frequent outcome.

Safe ways to remove wax

In such instances, first try to remove the wax by applying drops of a softening agent, several types of which are available without a prescription. One popular product contains hydrogen peroxide, which makes effervescent bubbles in the ear, softening and breaking loose the wax so that it will work its way out naturally. Other types are absorbed into the wax, softening it.

If the problem persists, many doctors recommend the use of a small syringe to irrigate the ear with warm water *(page 40)*. However, there is some danger of causing or spreading infection with this treatment. Even if no damage is done, irrigation sometimes can drive the wax deeper instead of flushing it out. In such cases, an ear specialist's ministrations may be needed. A doctor can see the problem better, can manipulate a syringe more skillfully and, if necessary, can bring other tools to bear. The implement physicians use most often is an ear speculum, a cone-shaped piece of metal with a hole at its tip. Inserted into the ear, the speculum pushes open and straightens the ear canal so that a tiny, shovel-like instrument can be inserted through its hollow tip to scoop out the plug of wax. Alternately, the physician may vacuum the wax out with a suction tube.

Any foreign substance that finds its way into the ear— from a drop of water to an insect or a button—can interfere with hearing. The first rule is: Remain calm. Despite the annoyance, resist the temptation to go fishing within the canal. The intruder can in most cases be removed by simple, safe measures.

If you get water in your ear, try lying on your side for a few moments, with the affected ear pointed down. If the droplet does not run out, you can experiment with the familiar poolside dance: Hop on the foot on the same side as the affected ear while cocking your head in that direction and gently tapping it, above the blocked ear, with the heel of your hand. A waterlogged ear may also be dried out by the use of alcohol drops, diluted with water to one-half strength; alcohol dissolves the trapped water, and the fluid then evaporates quickly. If these remedies fail to remove the water, it almost certainly will drain out as you move about during the day or as you sleep. Only if water remains in the ear for longer than 24 hours need you consult a physician, who can vacuum it out with his suction device.

Freeing the ears of foreign substances other than water is trickier. If an insect has flown or crawled into your ear, try any of these remedies:

● Pull on the flap of the outer ear—downward for children, up and back for adults; this sometimes straightens the canal sufficiently to let the creature fly or fall out.

● Hold an electric light just outside the ear. Most insects are attracted to light and so are lured out.

● While lying on the side opposite the affected ear, drip a small amount of warm baby oil or diluted alcohol into the ear. The intruder will drown in the warm liquid and fall out with a downward tilt of the head and ear.

If an inanimate object gets into an ear—as it often does in children, who are notorious for putting everything from erasers to peas into such openings—the only safe remedy is a downward pull on the ear flap while the head is shaken, ear pointed down. If this does not work, consult a physician. Do not flush the ear with water: The object may slide deeper into the ear canal and, if it is a porous material, may swell up and plug the passageway entirely. Similarly, do not try to extract the object with your fingers or with tweezers—you may drive it in deeper.

Flying without earaches

Among the natural materials that belong in the ear yet occasionally cause trouble, particularly during airplane flights, is air. "If the human ear was meant to fly," commented health writer Gloria Varley, "God shouldn't have given us Eustachian tubes." The Eustachian tubes are supposed to equalize the internal and external air pressure on the eardrum and thus allow the ears to adjust to rapid ascent or descent—whether in an airplane, elevator or automobile, or while diving in deep water.

Air occupies the middle ear. It gets there from the nose and mouth via the Eustachian tubes; a valve at the throat end of each tube regulates the flow, usually opening imperceptibly with every few swallows. When altitude changes, so does atmospheric pressure—falling with ascent, rising with descent. Normally the valve at the throat end of each Eustachian tube responds to this change in atmospheric pressure by opening automatically: The muscles involved react on cue to the pressure differential, and air rushes in or out to restore equilibrium.

Sometimes, however, the Eustachian tube will become clogged or swollen by a cold, an allergy, a sinus infection or some other ailment; then air cannot flow into or out of the middle ear to maintain pressure equilibrium. The high-pressure air on one side of the eardrum pushes the drum toward the low-pressure side. On ascent, the eardrum is pushed outward; on descent, inward. Pushed in either direction, it cannot respond to sound properly. The result is badly muffled hearing, ear pain and, sometimes, bleeding inside the ear. "Most doctors agree," said Dr. David N. F. Fairbanks of George Washington University recently, "that if you have an ear infection or cold in the early or acute phase, it's best not to fly."

If you cannot postpone your flight, however, there are several things you can do. If you have a cold, take a decongestant before and during the flight; it shrinks swollen tissues, widening the tubes. Next, try swallowing and yawning repeatedly; these mouth movements open the Eustachian tubes. If this does not clear the passage, chew a stick of gum, suck a mint or drink a glass of water. As a last resort, try the so-called Valsalva maneuver (named after Antonio Maria Valsalva, an Italian anatomist of the 17th Century): Take a mouthful of air, then pinch your nose shut with your fingers and close your mouth; next, gently try to force the air

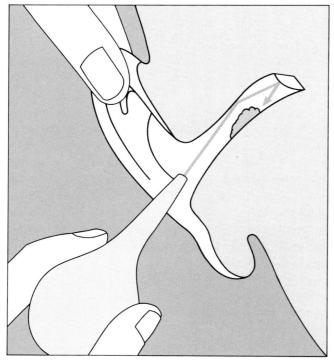

GETTING WAX OUT OF YOUR EARS
*Wax that interferes with hearing can usually be washed out
at home, as illustrated above. After softening the wax with drops
from the drugstore, fill a bulb syringe with water at or slightly
above body temperature. Lean over a wash basin, plugged ear
canted downward. Using the hand opposite the affected ear, reach
over the top of your head and gently pull the top of the ear up
and back. With your free hand, place the syringe, pointed slightly
upward, at the entrance to the ear canal; do not stick it in.
Squeeze gently, causing a stream of water to bounce off the top of
the ear canal and push the wax out from behind. If several
repetitions do not remove the wax, consult a doctor.*

out through your nose; when you hear a loud pop, you
have succeeded.

Babies are particularly prone to ear pain from clogged
Eustachian tubes during flight. To encourage swallowing
and the relief that comes with it, give the child a bottle of
water during ascent and descent.

Noise: an omnipresent danger

Dealing with air pressure, water in the ear or ear wax is
relatively simple. Easy-to-follow measures usually keep
trouble at bay. When problems occur, the symptoms generally are unmistakable and home remedies ordinarily effective.
Coping with another threat to the ears—noise—requires
more attention. Avoiding noise is sometimes impossible.
And because the damage it does usually occurs gradually,
detecting trouble is tricky.

As long ago as the First Century A.D., Pliny the Elder
reported that people living near a stretch of rapids on the Nile
River routinely became hard of hearing from the constant
roar of the waters. But excess noise was not a pervasive
problem until the Industrial Revolution. Then, in some tex-
tile centers in Scotland and England, it was not uncommon to
find virtually the entire working population of a town partially deaf from the sensory assault of the spinning frames and
looms. Such hazards were not confined to Britain: In 1882
Oscar Wilde was moved to write, ''America is the noisiest
country that ever existed. One is waked up in the morning not
by the singing of the nightingale but by the steel worker.'' He
went on to say that ''such continual turmoil must ultimately
be destructive.''

Noise, it is now realized, threatens people not only in the
industrial workplace but almost everywhere in the modern
world. The home throbs with the sound of a dozen machines
that grind, chop, wash, vacuum, dry, whip, compact and
dispose. Radios blare, motorcycles and trucks roar, ambu-
lances and police cars shriek, lawn mowers and chain saws
whine. Sports arenas, discotheques and video arcades can
prove even worse.

The intensity of sound—which determines its potential
for damage to hearing—is calculated in decibels (dB), a

term derived from the name of the acoustic theoretician and inventor of the telephone, Alexander Graham Bell. Zero decibels represents the faintest sound that can be heard by a normal human ear. This scale is logarithmic: Each decibel above zero represents not a simple numerical addition to intensity but a multiplication. An increase, say, from 60 decibels (the level of a normal conversation) to the 70 decibels typical of a loud restaurant is not one-sixth noisier but 10 times as noisy.

At 120 decibels most people with normal hearing begin to experience discomfort; subjected to noise levels between 130 and 140 decibels, they experience acute pain. Permanent damage can occur at levels much lower. Exposure to sounds of 115 decibels, even for a few seconds, will produce a tiny temporary hearing loss in some individuals, and prolonged, eight-hour-a-day exposure to noises in the 90-decibel range—not uncommon in the workplace—can result in permanent damage. The principal site of the damage is deep within the inner ear, where groups of the hair cells responsible for transmitting sound are vibrated so energetically by loud noise that they break.

Study after study bears out the damage that noise can do. In one unusual experiment led by Barbara A. Bohne of Washington University in St. Louis, six chinchillas were taken to a discotheque. Chinchillas were chosen not for their dancing ability but because their hearing sensitivity approximates that of humans. The animals were kept for more than two hours in a cage located a yard in front of a loudspeaker playing rock music as loud as 117 decibels. All of the chinchillas suffered ear damage.

The price exacted by discotheque din was measured in human terms in a recent study by Jane Madell of the New York League for the Hard of Hearing. She tested 70 discotheque disc jockeys, all under the age of 35. One third of them were found to have hearing that was significantly worse than average. "In that age group," she pointed out, "there shouldn't have been even one per cent with that kind of hearing loss."

The inescapable truth is that anyone who works or spends considerable time in a noisy environment can suffer noise-induced hearing loss. Tests of some 40 New York City firemen, all of whom had been exposed to siren noise for more than 10 years, revealed that 75 per cent had ear damage sufficient to impair hearing. Dentists, truck drivers, miners, machinists, foundry workers, shipbuilders and even farmers who ride tractors—all have been found in surveys to have substandard hearing.

Not surprisingly, people who spend their lives in hushed environments generally have superior hearing. In a 1960 study of the Central African Mabaan tribe, for example, researchers from Columbia University were astounded to find that the average Mabaan could discern a soft murmur across a clearing the size of a football field. The Mabaans lead a quiet life: The level of noise they meet with in their daily activities averages about one tenth that emitted by the average refrigerator. This helps explain why an 80-year-old Mabaan has better hearing than the average 30-year-old American.

Few people in the industrialized world can hope to live in as quiet an environment as the Mabaans do, although the law provides some workplace protection. In the United States, a federal regulation requires that constant noise levels for anyone working an eight-hour day not exceed 90 decibels. Exposure to higher noise levels is similarly regulated—no more than two hours a day at 100 decibels, 30 minutes at 110, and 15 minutes at 115.

Around the home, some commonsense measures can safeguard your hearing:

● Keep television sets, stereos and radios as low in volume as enjoyment will permit. Loudness is a habit that can be broken. Softer is safer.

● Do not run noisy household machines, such as the dishwasher (75 dB) and blender (88 dB), at the same time. Turn on the dishwasher only when you are ready to leave the kitchen, and if possible, shut the kitchen door.

● When operating noisy equipment such as lawn mowers, jig saws and chain saws, wear ear protectors, available at drug or hardware stores. A soft silicone earplug may screen out 15 to 35 decibels of excess noise, and an earplug of cotton wool soaked in paraffin can reduce noise levels by 20 to 30 decibels. Costlier, large ear muffs, the devices worn by ground personnel around airplanes, screen as much as 45 decibels of noise.

Treating infections

The ears, then, can be protected—if never wholly insulated—from noise, from the effects of fluctuating air pressure, and from disruptions caused by objects lodged in the canal. Other threats to hearing are subtler and can be countered only by a lifetime of vigilance and by prompt action when trouble flares. With proper care, infections can now be prevented or eliminated quickly, before they bring lasting harm. The effects of some common medicines must be monitored, so that their use can be discontinued if they cause ringing noises or other distortions of hearing. Some of the disorders that bear watching affect the outer ear, others the membrane—the eardrum—that separates it from the middle ear. Still others afflict the middle ear itself or the delicate structures of the inner ear. The deeper the trouble, the more serious it is. Indeed, many disorders of the inner ear are, for all practical purposes, incurable.

The outer ear, exposed to the environment, is often injured or attacked by disease, but because it is exposed its ills are generally simple to treat. It is susceptible to bacteria, particularly if scratched, and also to fungi, particularly if allowed to remain damp. One common infection promoted by dampness is called swimmer's ear, although its victims are not limited to those who swim. Anyone who lives in a warm, humid climate is at risk, leading the British to adopt another name for the condition: Hong Kong ear or Singapore ear, in not-so-fond memory of a hazard of colonial life in the Far East. By any name, it can be prevented by care in keeping the ears dry, and if contracted, it can be treated successfully with a nonprescription astringent known as Burow's solution. This remedy thwarts the fungal and bacterial growth of swimmer's ear by drying out and healing damp tissues, and at the

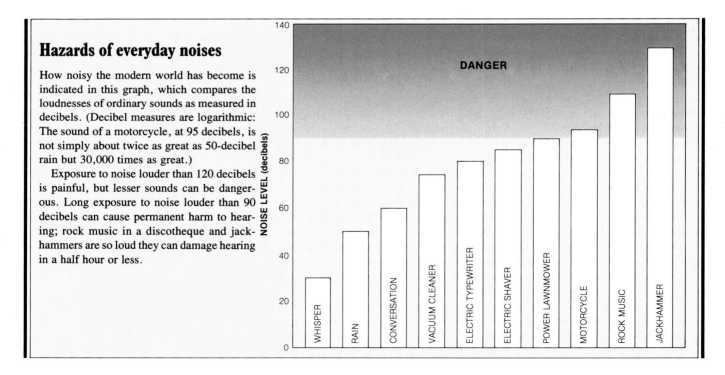

Hazards of everyday noises

How noisy the modern world has become is indicated in this graph, which compares the loudnesses of ordinary sounds as measured in decibels. (Decibel measures are logarithmic: The sound of a motorcycle, at 95 decibels, is not simply about twice as great as 50-decibel rain but 30,000 times as great.)

Exposure to noise louder than 120 decibels is painful, but lesser sounds can be dangerous. Long exposure to noise louder than 90 decibels can cause permanent harm to hearing; rock music in a discotheque and jackhammers are so loud they can damage hearing in a half hour or less.

NOISE LEVEL (decibels)

DANGER

WHISPER · RAIN · CONVERSATION · VACUUM CLEANER · ELECTRIC TYPEWRITER · ELECTRIC SHAVER · POWER LAWNMOWER · MOTORCYCLE · ROCK MUSIC · JACKHAMMER same time discourages reinfection by toughening the skin in the affected area.

More serious and more common are infections of the middle ear—otitis media, in medical jargon. They hurt, and they are dangerous, for they may damage the delicate parts of the hearing mechanism. The middle ear is susceptible because it is exposed, via the Eustachian tubes, to the variety of organisms that inhabit the nose and throat.

Under normal circumstances, a healthy Eustachian tube functions as a drainage pipe to rid the middle ear of fluids naturally secreted by the membranes lining its walls. In addition, defense mechanisms in the tubes keep infectious agents from getting into the middle ear. One part of the defense is mucus: It coats the tubes and traps foreign invaders, carrying them away as it flows down toward the throat. Another part of the defense is cilia: These tiny hairlike projections line the Eustachian tubes and move constantly in a waving motion, ensnaring germs and, in effect, sweeping them down the tubes and out into the throat. If cold, flu or strep-throat germs succeed in penetrating these defenses, though, and migrate into the middle ear through the Eustachian tubes, they can produce an infection that causes a rapid build-up of fluid in the cavity. At the same time, the Eustachian tubes swell, preventing drainage.

As fluid accumulates and the infection progresses, the eardrum turns red and bulges outward from the pressure, producing a severe earache and impaired hearing. The pain may radiate to the scalp and grow worse with the slightest tilt of the head. At this acute stage, without medical treatment the eardrum is likely to rupture within a few hours. Indeed, perforated eardrums from acute otitis media were quite common until after World War II, when penicillin and other antibiotics began to provide quick cures for such infections.

Ironically, the remarkable effectiveness of antibiotics has served to increase the incidence of another middle-ear disorder—serous otitis media, or fluid ear, which often follows an acute middle-ear infection. After bacteria have been routed by the antibiotics, the body fluids in which they were suspended stay behind, trapped temporarily by a still-swollen Eustachian tube. The fluids interfere with the movement of sound through the middle ear and usually cause some hearing loss. Serous otitis may clear up by itself, as the Eustachian tube returns to normal and allows the fluid to drain. Decongestants and antihistamines speed the return to normal, but in some cases surgery is needed to eliminate the fluid *(Chapter 5)*.

Middle-ear ailments and the aches and hearing loss they can bring afflict children more often than adults because of a quirk of anatomical development *(overleaf)*. An estimated 80 to 90 per cent of such disorders occur in children under the age of 12, and two thirds of all children suffer at least one bout before the age of three. Before long most children outgrow their susceptibility to earaches. As the years pass, other disorders begin to endanger hearing. Most of them—including immobilization of the ear bones and a mixed bag of defects lumped under the term presbycusis—were once blamed vaguely on the aging process. It now is becoming clear that they are brought on by a variety of causes, and they are not inevitable penalties of the passing years. Their impact can be blunted.

In the middle ear, the damage is done by otosclerosis, in which normal bone structure degenerates and is replaced by spongy tissue that eventually grows dense and hard, immobilizing the chain of tiny bones that transmits sound from the eardrum to the inner ear. Otosclerosis impairs hearing in approximately one out of every 100 people between the ages of 15 and 45. The condition is hereditary: In about 60 per cent of the cases, there is a family history of hearing difficulty; in 15 per cent of the cases, other family members are known to suffer from otosclerosis.

Otosclerosis primarily affects one bone in the chain, the stirrup, which is in contact with the inner ear. As the condition develops, spongy bone forms near the base of the stirrup. In most instances this growth is small and hearing disruption is minimal. But in some cases the soft tissue gradually covers the stirrup and hardens, freezing it to its inner-ear connection so that it cannot vibrate. Victims first lose sharpness in their hearing, generally in both ears. Faint sounds and low voices become hard to discern, then voices virtually disappear.

Certain drugs may slow this accretion of bone if used at the

How to spot an ear infection with an otoscope

An aching ear may feel bad all over, but the pain usually comes from an infection in one of two places—the external-ear canal, or the middle ear behind the eardrum. Signs of both types are easy to recognize if the family medical kit contains an otoscope, the magnifier-flashlight that doctors use to examine ears.

To check a sore ear, gently pull the flap back and up to straighten the passageway, as the mother shown below is doing. Then—very gently—insert the funnel-shaped viewing tip of the instrument and, while looking through the lens, direct the light down the canal leading to the eardrum and look for the reddish color of inflammation *(drawings, bottom)*. Evidence of infection should prompt an immediate call to the doctor.

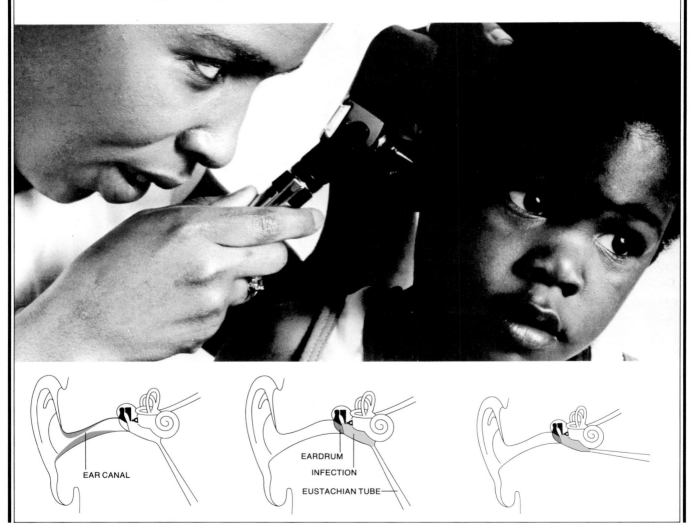

EAR CANAL

EARDRUM
INFECTION
EUSTACHIAN TUBE

EXTERNAL-EAR INFECTION
If an inflammation (red) is in the ear's outer canal, the canal appears swollen and pink or red in the light of the otoscope. The eardrum is usually unaffected and retains its normal pearly color.

MIDDLE-EAR INFECTION—ADULTS
The sign of an infected middle ear is a reddened eardrum, bulging with fluids. An adult ear generally resists infection because the Eustachian tube runs downward, aiding drainage.

MIDDLE-EAR INFECTION—INFANTS
In a child the signs of middle-ear infection are the same as in adults, but the affliction is more common: A more horizontal Eustachian tube conducts bacteria from the throat and drains fluids poorly.

first signs of hearing loss. High doses of sodium fluoride— the chemical that prevents tooth decay—appear to arrest the process by fostering the development of strong, dense bone cells, just as they harden tooth enamel. Sometimes the regimen is supplemented by calcium gluconate tablets or by other substances, such as vitamin D pills, that increase the fluoride's effectiveness. If drugs fail to arrest the disorder, delicate surgery can free the frozen bone.

What to do about ringing in the ears

One symptom of otosclerotic ear bones in the late stages of the disease is ringing—or buzzing, whistling, crackling, humming, roaring or hissing. But this so-called tinnitus, once dismissed by doctors as mysterious and untreatable, is now known to arise from a number of causes besides otosclerosis. Some can be avoided, others countered.

An estimated 36 million Americans hear the unwanted sounds of tinnitus, perhaps seven million of them so severely and persistently that they cannot lead normal lives. Jack A. Vernon of the University of Oregon was emphatic about its impact. ''I know of hardly anything,'' he said recently, ''that is more debilitating or robs the quality of life faster.'' For most victims the origin of the tinnitus is not in the middle ear but in the more delicate sensing structures of the inner ear and their connections to the brain.

Occasionally the troublesome sound is nothing more than the vibration of some part of the body—the rhythmic pulsing of blood or the clicking of a muscle in spasm. Even more rarely the ear itself emits noise, the sensors oscillating on their own to generate sounds that can sometimes be heard by other people nearby.

Most often, however, ringing is a perception of noises that are not there. It can be caused not only by otosclerosis but by mental stress, by an excess of fluid in the ear's balance organ or, in the majority of cases, by deterioration of the delicate, hairlike sensors.

Damage to these sensing cells can be caused by injury, such as a blow to the head or jaw, by nicotine in tobacco or caffeine in coffee, or by drugs such as aspirin, quinine, diuretics and antibiotics. Most doctors believe, however, that the greatest threat to the hair cells—and hence the most prominent cause of tinnitus—is noise. ''Hair cells simply aren't designed for the racket of modern civilization,'' said Vernon. ''You can walk on them a little and they spring back, but if you trample them too hard or too often, they flatten and die.''

Sensor damage might be expected to still sounds rather than create false sounds. One explanation of why the reverse can occur was offered by Vernon. ''We've known for years,'' he said, ''that hair cells produce electrical static, even when no sound is coming in. Your brain is used to ignoring this background noise.'' Yet if the hair cells are damaged, continued Vernon, there is ''no static from that region anymore. Your brain scans across, sees the empty spot, and says, 'Aha! Must be a signal!' In other words, your tinnitus may be the sound of silence.''

The best way to treat tinnitus is to address its suspected cause—avoiding noise, for example, or cutting down on aspirin or coffee. Some people can train their minds and bodies to relax on command, quieting tension-caused sound in the head. If the nonexistent noise cannot be turned off, it often can be overridden by a pleasant, low sound, such as a radio tuned to soft music—particularly useful at bedtime, when, in the quiet before sleep, tinnitus is most troublesome. Some people for whom tinnitus is a constant annoyance have even found relief through an electronic device that is worn like a hearing aid and emits a continuous masking signal.

The warning signs of deafness

Ringing in the ears is just one of the ear problems that may come with age. Noise, drugs, bone deterioration, nerve-cell degeneration, diminished blood circulation—all take their toll of hearing over the years.

Two out of every three people older than 65 suffer some degree of deafness: Voices become harder to hear, the television set must be played louder, the telephone bell sounds faint. In one out of every six cases, the impairment is significant enough to interfere with everyday communication. Its effect is so gradual that many victims do not notice their

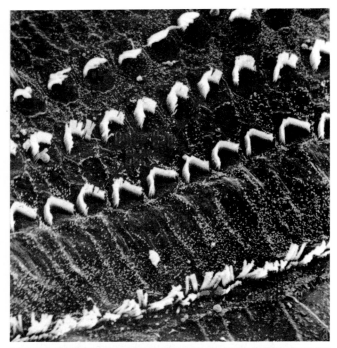

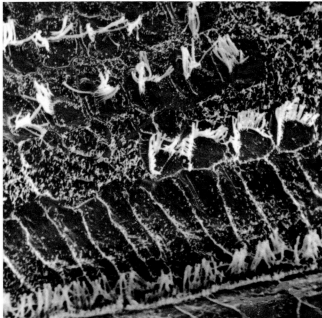

Damage done by noise is revealed in these electron micrographs comparing the inner ear of a normal guinea pig (top) with that of a guinea pig subjected for 24 hours to sound at the level of the loudest rock music. The noise has frayed and scarred three rows of the hair cells (seen here lined up across each picture) that must vibrate in response to sound waves.

difficulty (or, out of misplaced vanity, refuse to acknowledge it). Often a spouse or friend is the first person to detect the loss. Because so much can now be done to preserve or improve hearing, indications of approaching deafness should not be ignored, and it is useful to be alert for the signs. One way is to test yourself:

● Do you have to lean forward in order to hear what others are saying?

● Do you favor one ear over the other, unconsciously turning your head slightly to capture more sound?

● Do you have an easier time hearing men's conversation than women's and children's? (Response to the high-pitched tones in the voices of women and children generally is the first to fail.)

● Do you need to have sentences or words repeated?

● Do you routinely turn up the TV or radio to levels that cause others in the room to object?

● Do you find that background noise—in restaurants, parties, busy offices— makes it especially difficult for you to hear what others are saying?

● Do you increasingly decline social invitations because of the strain of maintaining conversation in gatherings?

● Do people, pets or cars seem to creep up on you without making a sound?

If the answer to several of these questions is "yes," you should have your hearing evaluated by a doctor. The doctor first will check to see that the trouble is not caused by something as simple as an obstruction. *The Australian Medical Association Gazette* recently reported the case of a 65-year-old patient who had gone to his physician with a complaint of longstanding hearing loss, convinced that he needed a hearing aid. Upon examination, the doctor discovered a curious obstruction in the ear. After removing it and questioning the patient, the doctor learned that, 60 years earlier, the patient had been treated for an infection by a doctor who had placed a cotton-wool plug in the boy's ear and told him to come back in a week. The boy and his mother forgot, and in time the plug became a permanent, sound-deadening fixture.

Not many people allow an obstruction to go unnoticed for 60 years, but the seemingly elementary procedure of looking into the ear canal often does yield dramatic results. Some people think they are going deaf, when in fact their only problem is excess ear wax.

After visual inspection of the ear, most doctors make a simple assay of hearing sensitivity with a tuning fork *(page 37)*. A more thorough evaluation requires the expertise and equipment of specialists: either an otolaryngologist (a physician trained to treat the ear, nose and throat) or an otologist (an ear specialist). These physicians may in turn call upon an audiologist, a professional in hearing measurement.

How hearing is tested

The experts first seek to learn the character of the hearing loss. They may make a rough determination with tuning forks. For more precise tests, however, the diagnostician will rely on a pure-tone audiometer, a device that electronically produces tones similar to those made by tuning forks. Each tone consists of a single pitch, which is indicated by the frequency of vibration of the sound wave, measured in hertz. (This measure, synonymous with the older term ''cycles per second,'' honors the discoverer of radio waves, German physicist Heinrich Hertz.)

The patient usually sits in a soundproof cubicle, first wearing earphones, then wearing an electrical vibrator that presses against the skull behind the ear to test the conduction of sound through bone directly to the inner ear. During the earphone test, the examiner turns on one tone at a time, beginning with the tenor note of 125 hertz and ranging upward to a shrill 8,000 hertz. Each tone is directed first into one ear, then the other. Initially, the tones are played so softly they are inaudible; then they are increased in loudness by measured steps until the subject signals that he can just barely hear the tone. The tester follows this procedure for each pitch in turn, repeating the sequence from soft to loud until the subject responds. The loudness (measured in decibels) required to make audible each pitch (indicated in hertz) is then plotted on a graph.

The average child can hear all the tones in the range, from a low of 20 hertz to a high of about 20,000 hertz—more than six octaves above middle C on the piano. This magnificent range of response shrinks gradually thereafter even in healthy adults, however, as age diminishes the ear's ability to pick up the higher tones *(overleaf)*.

Tests that involve pure tones indicate the patient's sensitivity to sound, but do not necessarily reveal how well he actually hears, that is, how well his hearing mechanism responds to spoken language. To account for this, ear specialists nowadays conduct a test involving the words of normal speech. At various decibel levels, a series of common one- and two-syllable words—an, us, what, birthday, cowboy, toothbrush—is played to the patient, who is asked to identify what he hears. Ultimately, the examiner establishes the levels at which the spoken words are barely audible, most comfortable and uncomfortably loud.

Such tests usually uncover one of the two basic kinds of hearing loss. The simpler category, called conductive loss, involves a fault in the mechanical transmission of sound, mainly in the middle ear; it is this type that is associated with damage to the eardrum, fluid in the middle ear, and most cases of otosclerosis. Conductive hearing loss muffles all sounds, and in severe cases, makes sounds softer than around 60 decibels difficult to hear. At levels above 60 decibels, however, sounds can bypass the middle ear; skull bones pick up the vibrations and transmit them to the inner ear.

The second major category of hearing loss arises in the inner ear, from a malfunction affecting either the hairlike sound receptor cells or the auditory nerve itself. Most people who are born with impaired hearing suffer from this so-called sensorineural hearing loss, but such impairment is also brought on by age, noise, drugs, chemicals and tumors.

Unlike conductive loss, which deprives the ears of the ability to hear all sounds at their full level, sensorineural loss affects response at certain pitches. The receptors sensitive to high notes usually degenerate first. This alteration in the sound spectrum brings a number of inconvenient consequences. Vowels, which generally are below 1,000 hertz, may be heard clearly, but consonants, most of higher pitch, appear to drop out of words. For the same reason, the voices of women and children, usually higher in pitch than men's voices, may become harder to hear. Even birdwatching is

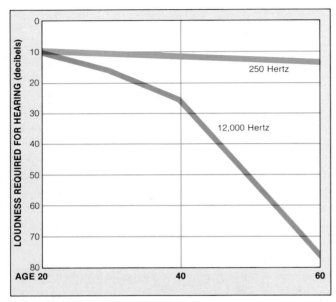

HOW HEARING FADES WITH AGE
Though advancing years bring diminished sensitivity to all sounds, the ability to hear high-pitched sounds drops off much more than responsiveness to low pitches (graph above). At the age of 20 the average person can hear a sound of any pitch at a loudness of 10 decibels—far fainter than a whisper. Thereafter sensitivity to low-pitched sounds, such as those measured as 250 hertz (blue, middle C on the piano), remains fairly constant. However, for a 60-year-old a note of 12,000 hertz (red, five and a half octaves above middle C) has to be louder than 70 decibels to be heard.

affected. One dedicated bird watcher found that as he grew older the high-pitched call of the blue-winged warbler became faint while the full-throated song of the cardinal remained clear as ever.

Some people suffer from both major types of deafness. A few individuals lose their hearing although there is nothing physically wrong with their ears or their nerves. Such ''functional'' loss is psychological in origin. In one dramatic case, a New York mother of a handicapped boy lost her hearing abruptly. Yet examination found her ears normal, and her acoustic reflex—a muscular contraction that can be detected when loud noises bombard the middle ear—was acceptable. Only after deeper inquiry was an answer found: The mother's overstressed mind had devised deafness as a means of escape. Psychiatric counseling soon restored her hearing.

Although hearing lost to conductive disorders can be fully restored by surgery in some cases, in other cases the operation leaves hearing incomplete. For those with sensorineural loss, surgery is not yet of much help. Thus a victim of either type of deafness may need a hearing aid.

Getting the right hearing aid

The modern hearing aid works like a miniature public address system to amplify sounds so that they can be heard. It has a microphone to catch sounds approaching the ear and change them into electrical impulses, an amplifier to magnify those impulses, and an earphone to convert the amplified impulses back into sound, which then enters the ear.

Thanks to transistors, hearing aids can be made small enough to fit inside an ear button. This type, combining microphone, amplifier and earphone in a single unit, is almost invisible, but does not provide enough power to help people who have more than moderate hearing loss. And its extremely small size makes changing batteries difficult for those with arthritic fingers or limited vision.

The majority of the aids used today are the behind-the-ear type: A small flesh-colored case about the size of a plump pea pod fits snugly into the niche between the external ear and the skull; it sends amplified sound through a crook-shaped tube to a plug in the ear canal. An even less obtrusive version is built into the temples of eyeglass frames. (A few people so dislike the image of the hearing-aid wearer that they choose the more discreet eyeglass type even though they do not need glasses.)

A specialized application of eyeglass-frame aids is the CROS system, an acronym for "contralateral routing of signals." It involves putting a microphone over an ear with poor hearing and routing the sound signals around, through the frames, to the other, better ear. This technique strengthens hearing and also gives the wearer some indication of the direction of sound because it delivers sounds from the side that would ordinarily be silent.

A type of hearing aid that has its microphone and amplifier in a pocket-sized case worn around the body provides the greatest assistance of all. Because the less conspicuous types have been improved, this around-the-body aid is not needed for most adults. However, it is generally prescribed for a deaf child for pragmatic reasons: It is less likely to be lost, it is more durable, and its controls are easier to operate.

Getting the right hearing aid is much more difficult than being fitted with eyeglasses, because ear tests, unlike the measurements of eye defects, give only indirect clues to a remedial prescription. Hearing examinations primarily determine thresholds: the softest sounds that are just barely audible. The ability to hear louder sounds may be quite different, and it is the louder-than-threshold sounds that people most often want to hear.

Despite such limitations, hearing tests help the doctor set basic requirements for a hearing aid suited to an individual's impairment. The device must amplify sounds enough to bring thresholds to normal levels but not so much that sounds are uncomfortably loud; and it must do so over the tonal range of normal speech, about 300 to 3,000 hertz. These basic requirements are only a guide; in the end the hearing aid is chosen by trial and error, sometimes with the help of a master aid, a special instrument that can be adjusted to mimic the qualities of many different commercial hearing aids. The selection should be made with the guidance of a doctor, not solely on the advice of a hearing-aid dealer. The characteristics of makes and models vary widely, and the doctor can

prescribe any of the hundreds on the market; a dealer's choice may be much more limited.

Although choosing a hearing aid requires close collaboration between doctor and patient, adjusting to it is essentially an individual matter. "Getting your first hearing aid is a lot like getting your first bicycle," said one wearer. "You expect to be able to take it out for a spin the minute you get your hands on it, but as I discovered to my chagrin, it takes a lot of scrapes and bruises and someone running alongside offering encouragement before you can ride away in confidence." It takes several visits to the doctor and a good deal of practice, in fact, before instrument and wearer are working together satisfactorily.

Hearing aids are no more a panacea than the other remedies for deafness. Some types of hearing loss are not helped by amplification. And in other types the loss may be so profound that sound cannot be amplified to a level that will make normal conversation accessible. Such people must learn to supplement whatever sound they are able to receive electronically by "hearing" with their eyes. Although everyone who can see unconsciously supplements hearing by reading lips and facial expressions when in conversation with others, the technique can be refined to a reasonably effective skill with training and practice.

Visual and even tactile substitutes for hearing are particularly important to deaf or hearing-impaired children if they are to learn to speak and communicate effectively with others. But such aids cannot be brought to bear until the problem is diagnosed: Early detection of hearing loss is crucial. A child who does not react to the sound of a rattle by the age of six or nine months should be tested by an ear specialist. If hearing loss is found, prompt treatment and special training can help the child overcome a handicap that, without expert attention, might prove overwhelming.

For everyone, young and old, the communication afforded by language, principally by way of the ear, remains the crucial human skill. Thanks to modern knowledge of the mechanism of hearing and new techniques for treating its ills, this essential sense can now be protected, preserved and repaired far better than ever before. ✳

Teaching deaf children to make themselves heard

Deafness is a handicap to anyone, but to children under the age of three it can be disastrous. Few such youngsters live in a world of total silence; most can hear some sounds with hearing aids. Yet many are so severely impaired that, unless they are given intensive special training, they cannot learn to use the currency of normal communication: the spoken word. ''No one really appreciates the nature of the handicap,'' said the father of a deaf son. ''The problem is not that these children can't hear, but that they can't learn language.''

Hampered in the ability to manage this conventionally— that is, by hearing words and imitating them—deaf children must be taught to communicate in some other fashion. Otherwise they are essentially lost to human society.

Educators differ bitterly on how best to help deaf children break the sound barrier. Some believe that deaf youngsters must be taught to communicate with their voices; others urge the hand and arm signals of sign language. The controversy has raged for more than a century.

On one side are the disciples of Thomas Hopkins Gallaudet, the New Englander who, in the early 19th Century, traveled to France to learn sign language at a pioneering Parisian school for the deaf, then brought the method back home. Gallaudet considered vocal training for the deaf a parlor trick, ''entitled,'' he said, ''to rank little higher than training starlings or parrots.'' Even after much time and effort, the results of vocal training are limited. By the age of five, for example, a deaf child trained from infancy may be able to produce some 200 words, compared with 5,000 to 20,000 for a child with hearing. Using gestures instead of the voice, a deaf child can learn to express more ideas at an earlier age.

Opposing Gallaudet's philosophy are experts who argue that sign language is a linguistic crutch dooming a deaf person to life in a silent subculture. These educators insist that deaf children should rely entirely on speech and lip reading; sign language is prohibited in their classrooms.

The debate continues, but since the early 1970s, many training centers, such as Kendall Demonstration Elementary School in Washington, D.C., have adopted a hybrid method, called total communication. It not only combines instruction in speech and lip reading with training in sign language, but also teaches students to use mime, gestures, body language and touch—in short, to take advantage of every possible skill of perception and expression that can help them communicate with one another and with a hearing world.

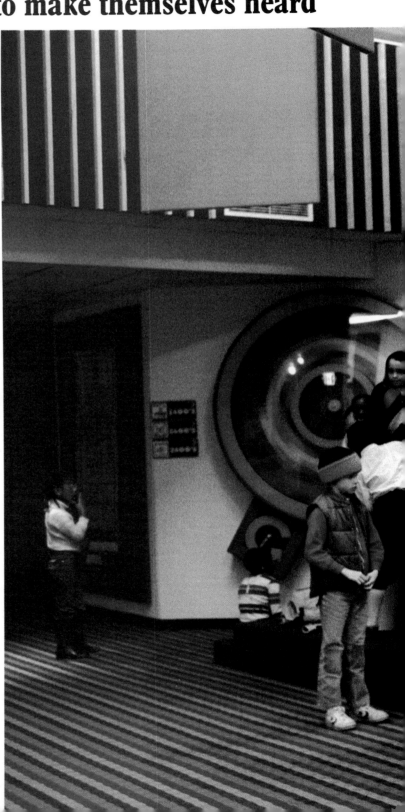

As the school day begins, students assemble in Kendall School's central hallway, greeting friends and playing with large wall-mounted, pinball-like games. In the foreground, two girls, wearing powerful aids that help them make use of what hearing they have, perch on the edge of the platform and hold an animated conversation in sign language.

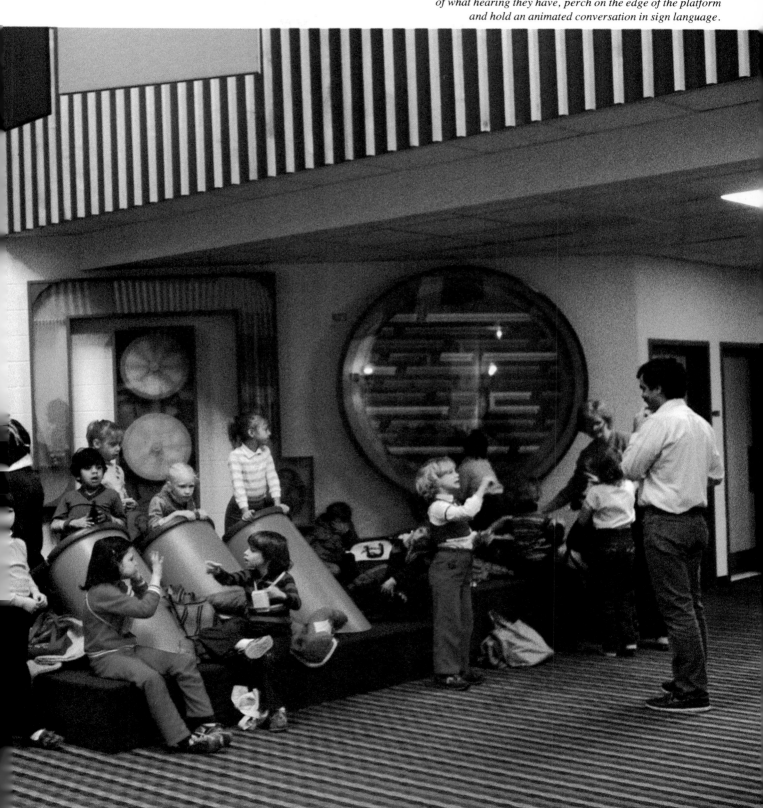

*Three-year-old Danny McComas adjusts the earpiece of the
Phonic Ear that is strapped to his chest for the day; his regular
hearing aid is in a picture-identified pouch of the wall hanging.
The helmet protects Danny in falls due to poor coordination—
a legacy, like his deafness, of a meningitis infection.*

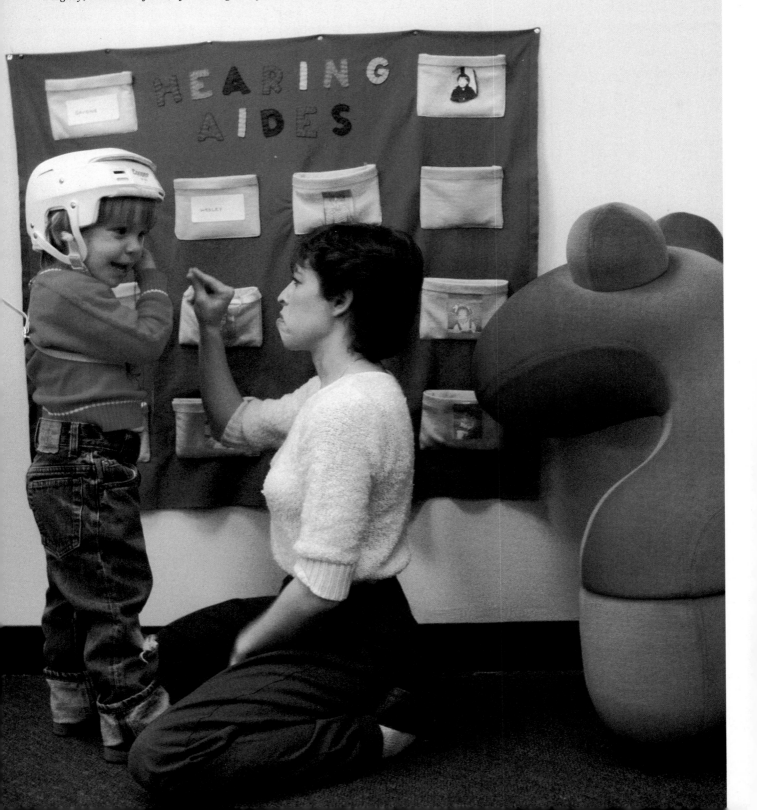

Making use of minimal hearing

Because most deaf children possess at least some ability to detect sound, the Kendall School's first step is to help them make use of what hearing they have. To that end, audiologists—experts who test hearing—evaluate each pupil repeatedly.

About half of the students at Kendall can hear no sound softer than 90 decibels—the equivalent of a shout from a foot away. Yet any hearing, however substandard, can be useful in learning. Thus, almost all students wear individually tailored hearing aids. During school time many pupils replace these aids with special devices that enable them to concentrate more easily on their classwork. Known by one of their trade names, Phonic Ear, they combine hearing aids with short-range radios. The voice of a teacher speaking into a microphone is broadcast to receivers strapped to the students' chests, and from there wires take it directly to the children's ears, eliminating background noise.

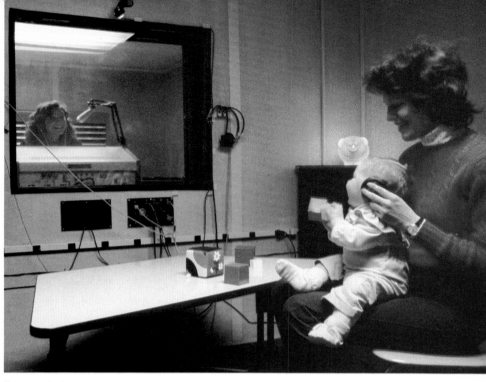

To test a baby's hearing, an audiologist lights a toy pig (background) while sending a tone to headphones the mother holds. Next, she will see if a softer tone—and no light—also makes the baby look at the pig.

While his teacher watches, a three-year-old listens through his hearing aid for a tone signaling him to drop a block into a can. The audiologist will repeat the test with different aids so she can select the best for him.

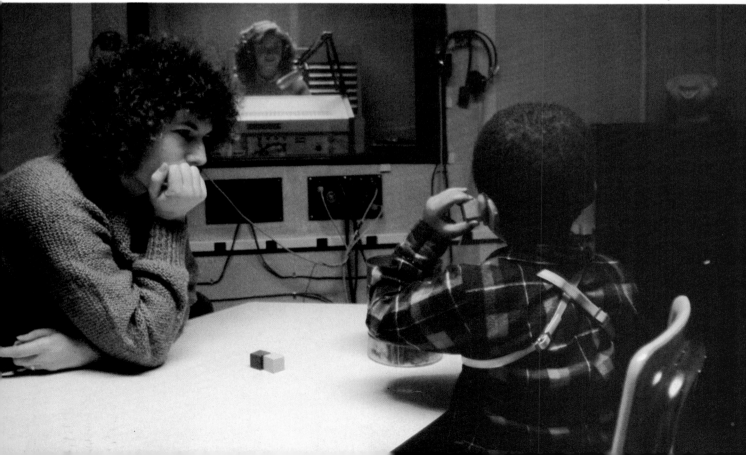

Communicating in mixed media

Children at Kendall School are encouraged to use all of the sensory resources at their command. Classes are taught not only in speech —which the children both lip-read and hear in fragments through hearing aids—but also in three sign languages, informal gestures and mime. Teachers speak and sign simultaneously; most children prefer to use American Sign Language, the swiftest and most idiomatic of the three systems they learn.

"Ameslan" uses about 6,000 signs, with grammar and syntax often quite unlike that of spoken English. For example, Ameslan for "I didn't give the teacher a Christmas gift" comes out as "Teach-person, not to-give-a-gift, Christmas"; one sign stands for "to give a gift," and "teacher" is represented by the signs for "teach" and "person."

In order to understand standard English, students learn signed English, which uses signs in regular sentence order. Finally, they learn to spell words out with their fingers.

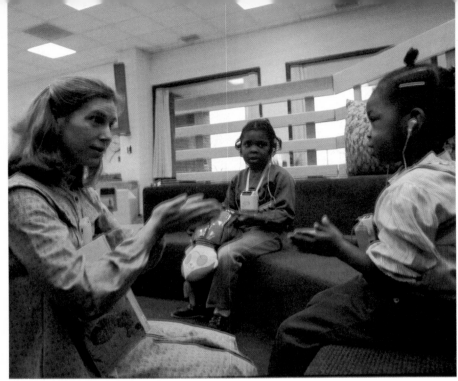

A teacher shows a child the sign for "book" (above) and simultaneously says the word, so that the four-year-old will learn that the sign, the lip movements and the few sounds she can hear all have the same meaning.

A language specialist asks an eight-year-old to arrange blocks in a specific order. Later, the partition on the table is removed so that the child can compare his stack with hers and see how well he understood.

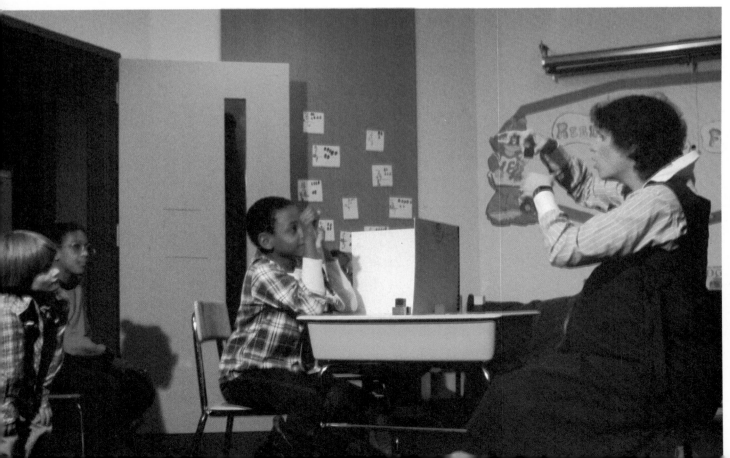

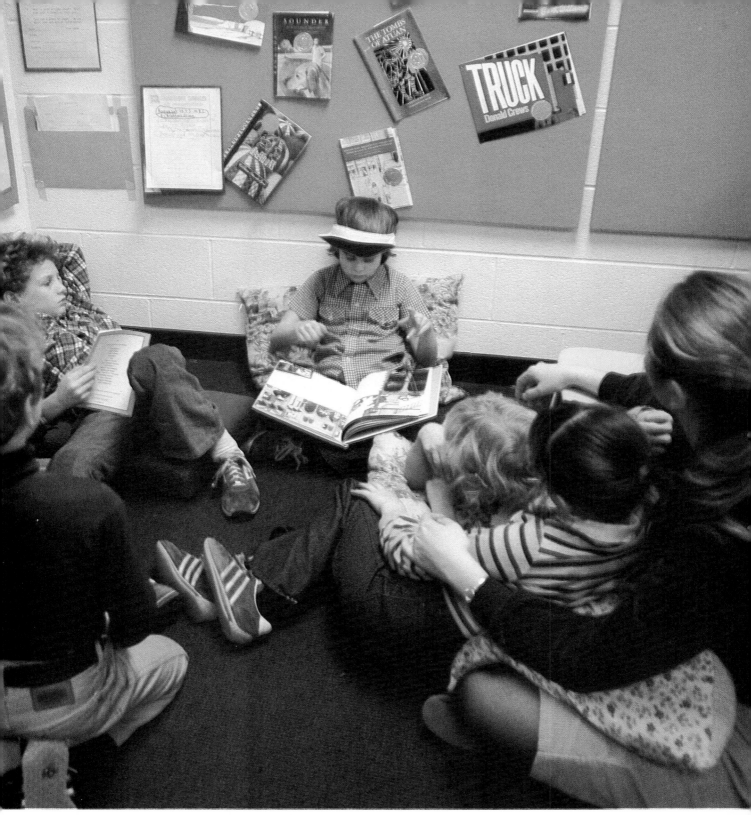

At the end of the day, pupils sprawl comfortably on the floor as
a classmate reads to them, translating a storybook tale into signs.
Unlike some 95 per cent of deaf children, these six- to eight-
year-olds have deaf parents; taught sign language from infancy,
they are far more fluent than most deaf children their age.

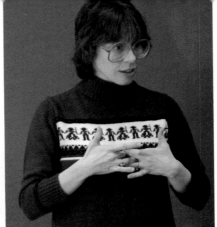

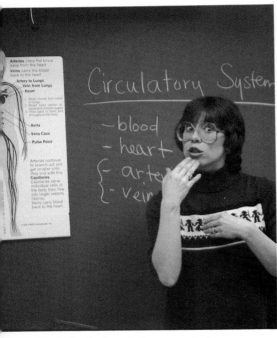

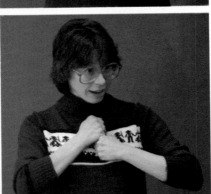

Using four Ameslan signals, from top to bottom at left, the teacher explains the basic fact of blood circulation to her class.

THE HEART

PUMPS

At the beginning of a lesson on the human circulatory system, a teacher signs the word ''good'' to students who have just mastered the signals for the four key words written on the chalkboard behind her. Most hand symbols in American Sign Language take about twice as long to produce as spoken words. But because the signs can compress several words into one gesture—as illustrated at right— lessons can be taught at a brisk pace.

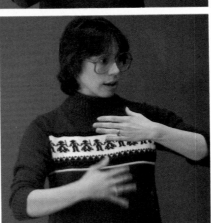

BLOOD

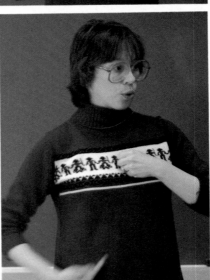

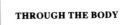

THROUGH THE BODY

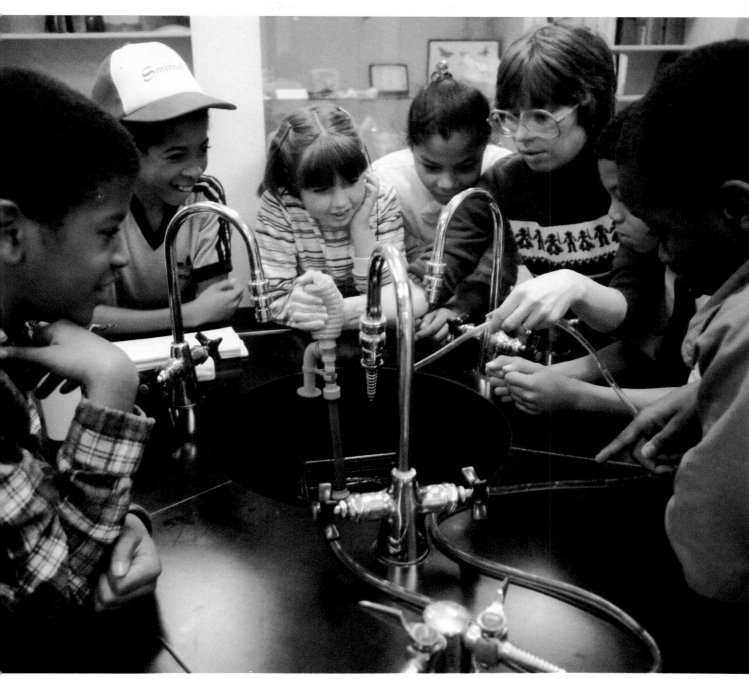

To aid comprehension of the just-completed lesson on the circulatory system, the class gathers around a laboratory sink for a demonstration: The teacher simulates the functions of the heart and blood vessels by squeezing a plastic bellows that pumps colored liquid through a clear tube.

Learning to shape the sounds of speech

Deaf children rarely have anything wrong with their vocal cords. Yet they encounter two enormous difficulties in learning to use this apparatus: Unable to hear others clearly, they lack a good model for speech; unable to hear themselves very well, they cannot shape sounds into subtle speech patterns.

To overcome these obstacles, teachers turn noisemaking into a kind of game. In daily practice, the children move their lips and tongues and vibrate their vocal cords to produce sounds that are made perceptible to sight or touch by a variety of devices. Some are as simple as a feather *(right)*. Others use microphones and electronic circuits to activate vibrators, turn on a light or generate patterns indicating tone on a display screen *(opposite)*.

In this way a student learns to produce a variety of sounds and to vary them in pitch and volume. In the next stage the child acquires a repertoire of vowels and consonants; the consonants are particularly troublesome to learn, since they are generally high-pitched —the very tones that most hearing-impaired people have the greatest difficulty picking up. But once children can produce individual sounds at will, they can try for the goal: assembling sounds into words.

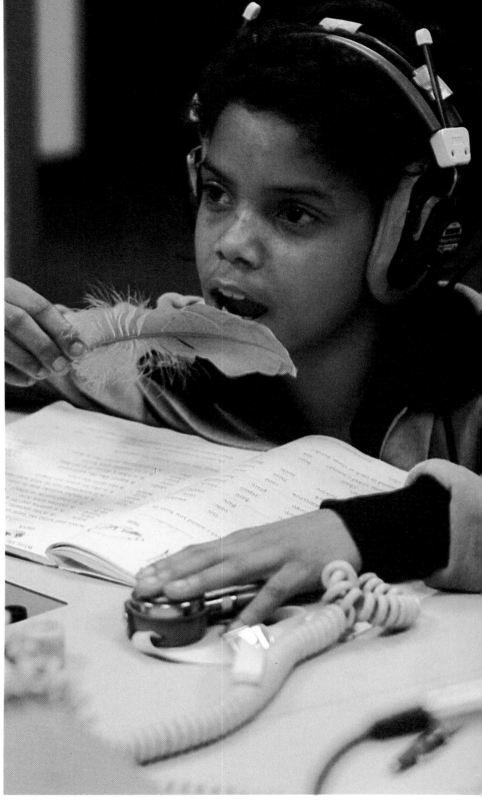

Reading out loud from a workbook, a 13-year-old uses sight, touch and his own minimal hearing to improve his speech. He watches a feather respond to puffs of air produced by ''f'' and ''s'' sounds; a device under his left hand translates the sounds he makes into vibrations he can feel, while his headphones bring the amplified tones of his own voice to his ears.

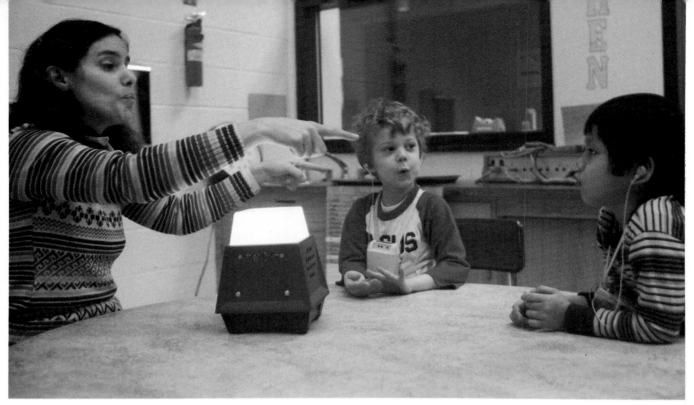

Imitating the facial movements of their teacher, students wearing Phonic Ears produce sounds that activate the noise-sensitive light on the table. The children learn to associate the brightness of the light with the loudness and duration of the sounds they make.

A four-year-old girl, responding to her teacher's raised-arm signal, enunciates a vowel into a microphone device that changes sound into a pattern on the screen. The spidery pattern is characteristic of the ''ah'' sound she was asked to make.

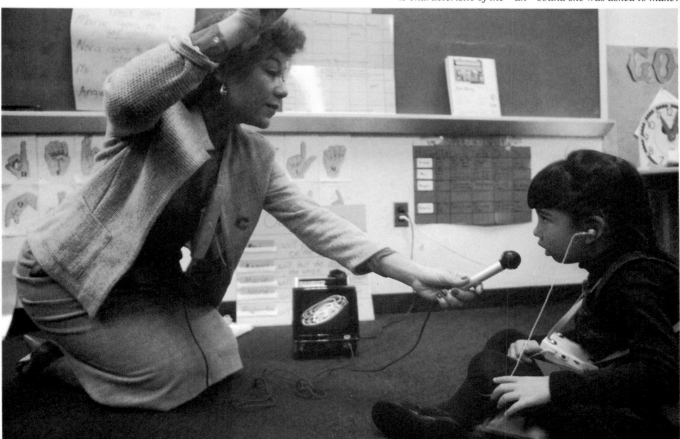

The goal: a full life

By the time they finish Kendall School at the age of 15, most students are able to express themselves fluently in sign language, and many have acquired a basic command of spoken English. With language as a foundation, they can study literature, mathematics and social and physical sciences. They participate in athletics and are exposed to music *(right)*, even though they may not hear much of it.

To the extent possible, their education parallels that of hearing children, although they lag several grade levels behind their hearing counterparts. From Kendall Elementary School, most of the students go on to a special secondary school, and some eventually enroll in college. Able to communicate—not only with one another, but with hearing people as well—deaf children no longer need live in a world that is radically circumscribed by their handicap.

After a concert by Officer Friendly's Side by Side Band—a musical group sponsored by the local police department—children crowd onto the Kendall auditorium's stage to examine the instruments and meet the performers. Even though deaf children can hear few musical notes, they easily feel the rhythmic vibrations produced by loud brass and percussion instruments.

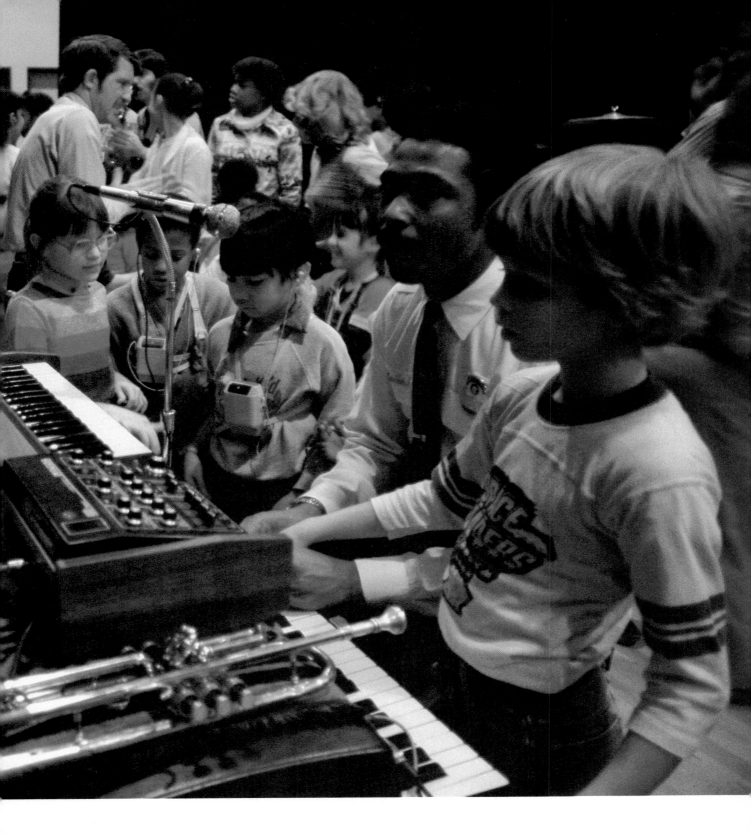

CHAPTER 3

Remedies for eye complaints

How to prevent eyestrain
Causes and cures of inflammation
When to take an eye exam—and from whom
What the charts tell
Getting the right glasses
Pros and cons of contact lenses

A newborn baby comes into the world equipped with a superb pair of eyes—but can barely see. The infant can tell the difference between light and dark, and can make out bulky forms, but cannot by sight distinguish mother from father. Gradually—far more gradually than most parents realize—discrimination of shapes and colors is refined, sight becomes more acute and the child masters the art of three-dimensional vision. Vision continues to improve as it is used more intensively and for a greater variety of purposes until, during the teens, a kind of stable maturity takes hold. In most ways and for most people, the eyes are then working as well as they ever will.

Over the years a host of minor eye disturbances may interfere with comfortable seeing for a time. Many of these problems can be prevented and most can be treated at home or cured by properly fitted eyeglasses. Children with colds have inflamed, watery eyes; teen-age girls are prey to eye infections that are spread by shared cosmetics; both girls and boys turn up with black eyes from time to time, or contract conjunctivitis, sties and eyestrain. In adolescence permanent defects of vision, due to slight malformations of the eyeball or the cornea, make their appearance.

By the age of 21, about 35 per cent of all Americans are troubled by nearsightedness, approximately 60 per cent are farsighted and at least one third require prescriptions for the distortions known as astigmatism. By middle age, a universal imperfection—presbyopia, which is a decreasing ability to focus on near objects—develops; by the fifties, for nearly everyone, the arms are not long enough to hold a book where the words can be distinguished, and bifocals or reading glasses generally become indispensable. At all ages eyestrain brings pain and fatigue.

None of these conditions need be dangerous. Still, there is no reason you should put up with their discomforts. Once you learn how to arrange lighting and seating for close work, when to wear sunglasses and how to rest your eyes, you can avoid the aches of eyestrain. Similarly, a few simple rules of hygiene and basic home remedies will ease the common eye ailments. And understanding when—and why—glasses should be prescribed will help you keep your vision comfortably sharp over the years.

There are few misconceptions about health that are more firmly rooted than those relating to eyestrain. When Grandmother warned, ''You'll ruin your eyes reading in that dim light,'' she was wrong, at least in a technical sense. You cannot damage your eyes merely by working in dim (or bright) light. Nevertheless, Grandmother was right in issuing a caution: You can get the heavy eyelids, irritation and headache of eyestrain by using poor light.

What constitutes ''poor light'' is equally misunderstood. Indeed, you are less likely to get eyestrain by reading in dim light than in bright light that is misdirected. Yet the causes of eyestrain are simple and so are the preventives and remedies.

Eyestrain is generally some kind of strain of the many muscles in the eye or associated with it. Some of these muscles control the up, down and sideways movement of the

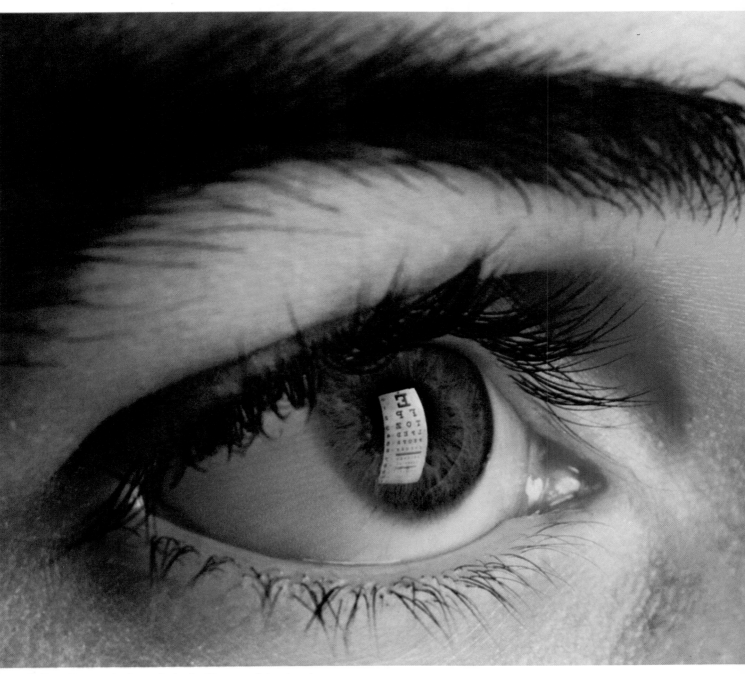

*Reflected in a patient's eye is the familiar test of visual acuity,
a version of the chart devised in 1864 by Dutch ophthalmologist
Herman Snellen. Each line is rated according to the distance
at which it could be read by someone with normal sight. Someone
with 20/200 vision can read, from 20 feet away, only the lines a
normally sighted person distinguishes at 200 feet.*

eyeball, others pull on the ligaments holding the lens to change its shape for focusing, and others open and narrow the iris to adjust the amount of light the pupil admits. Although all of these muscles work uncomplainingly while you are awake (and even while you sleep), they can be fatigued by extraordinary demands. For example, looking up repeatedly from a shaded book on the beach to watch a child in the water is very likely to give you tired eyes, as muscles must not only move the eye but try to help it adapt to large, sudden changes in illumination. Even worse stress is placed on the muscles when they must hold the eyes in one position for a long time; driving for hours with eyes locked in focus on the road ahead will cause eye fatigue, and so will reading for hours with eyes locked in focus on the nearby page.

Close work in dim light results in muscle fatigue because precise sight requires enough illumination to produce contrast between details in the work. To make up for the lack of clarity in dim light, most people hold the work very close so that it appears larger, thus straining the focusing muscles. The focusing muscles tire, too, if they continually try to clarify an image blurred by eyes that need glasses (or a new prescription).

Very bright light, such as the glaring reflection off a wet road or a glossy magazine page, strains the muscles trying to narrow the pupil and may also cause squinting, which fatigues other muscles. More troublesome is excessive contrast—a spot of bright illumination surrounded by darkness or vice versa—which causes contradictory signals to be sent to the eye controls. Flicker, such as that produced by malfunctioning fluorescent lamps, television sets or computer screens, has a similar effect.

Some causes of eyestrain appear to have no connection to the eyes. Many drugs—including commonly prescribed diarrhea medicines—so increase sensitivity to light that dark glasses may be necessary for comfort out of doors even when the sky is overcast. Posture, too, is surprisingly important. Reading in bed or in a very soft chair for a long period of time can lead to slouching with neck bent, eyes held in an unnatural position, and tension throughout the head and the muscles of the eyes. Slouchers who wear glasses may also

lose the advantages of seeing through the centers of their lenses; instead, they are likely to look through the somewhat distorting margins.

How to prevent eyestrain

To avoid eyestrain, make things easy for your eyes:

● Illuminate work brightly. A 100-watt incandescent (or 20-watt fluorescent) bulb in a desk or floor lamp usually suffices; ideally it should shine over your shoulder (the left one if you are right-handed). Translucent lampshades that are open at the top are best because they distribute the light around the room. If you must rely on a ceiling fixture, bear in mind that doubling the distance to the light source necessitates a four-fold increase in illumination. And old people require more illumination than young ones because of a number of anatomical changes brought about by age: The normally transparent parts of the eye become less transparent, the iris stiffens so that it cannot open so wide, and the retina loses some of its sensitivity to light.

● Illuminate the room fairly brightly to eliminate strain-causing contrasts. Do not try to work in a small pool of bright light in a darkened room.

● Arrange seating and work surface so that you do not need to bend your head or lean over to see clearly. Reading material should be held at a 45° angle to the table, about 14 inches from the eyes; for reading at a desk, a small, angled easel is useful. To read in bed, sit up.

● Rest your eyes at least every 20 minutes. Look up from close work so that you refocus on distant objects; when driving, glance occasionally to the side of the road or to the instrument panel.

● Change the position of your body every hour or so. Stand up, stretch, take a few deep breaths and walk around. Driving is much less fatiguing if you stop every few hours and get out of the car for some exercise.

● Make sure the work is stationary and sharp. Adjust the viewing screen of a television set or computer terminal so that the image is clear and flicker is eliminated. Do not try to read or sew in a moving car.

● Wear tinted glasses and a brimmed hat in bright sunlight.

Polarizing spectacles help to reduce the glare reflected from snow and water.

Even maximum prudence cannot always prevent eyestrain. When it develops, one remedy is certain: rest. The irritation and headache should disappear in an hour or so. Recovery can be speeded by the prescription that Dr. Ben Esterman, a noted American eye doctor, worked out in medical school when "more study was necessary and it was already past 2 a.m." His treatment consists simply of hot and cold compresses applied alternately to the closed eyelids for four or five minutes. The sudden changes of temperature stimulate circulation and allay fatigue; they are, as Dr. Esterman pointed out, "similar to the cold shower and rubdown between the halves of a football game."

Getting the red out

Victims of eyestrain in many cases have bloodshot eyes—a general redness caused by blood vessels that are swollen, carrying an increased flow of blood to the tired eyes. Bloodshot eyes can result not only from strain but also from the inflammation of conjunctivitis, alcohol consumption, sleeplessness, and the irritation generated by cigarette smoke, dust or chemical pollutants.

Generally no more than a temporary annoyance, bloodshot eyes heal themselves as rest returns blood vessels to normal size. Yet an extraordinary number of people will not let well enough alone. About a third of the medicines used on the eyes are over-the-counter preparations designed to remove redness and relieve soreness.

Treatments for these ailments are traditional all over the world, and some of the simplest probably work as well as any. Among the folk remedies are poultices of raw cucumber slices or cold tea bags; they make the patient close and rest his eyes and they ease discomfort as their coolness constricts blood vessels. But some old mixtures seem less likely to help. Here is a prescription for "EYE, or EYELIDS inflamed" from the medical section of *Consult Me,* a popular home reference published in 1872: "Apply as a poultice, boiled, roasted, or rotten apples warm.—Or, wormwood tops with the yolk of an egg. This will hardly fail."

Allowing time to see in the dark

People, like cats, have an admirable ability to see both in the dark and in bright light. But adjustment to abrupt changes in lighting takes time, and eyes may be left temporarily—sometimes dangerously—helpless until the adaptation process is complete.

The time lag for vision in the dark is most pronounced when illumination decreases suddenly; a few moments of nearly total blindness are followed by half an hour or more of diminished vision. Stepping briskly at night from a lighted cabin onto a wooded path invites a fall, and driving from a lighted city street onto an unlighted road makes most people suddenly unable to see pedestrians or bicyclists at the side of the pavement.

The reason for the slow adaptation to darkness lies in the way the eye works. The retina sends a nerve signal when light bleaches pigments in the rod and cone cells, changing the chemical form of the pigments. In their changed form, they are no longer sensitive to light; the body must regenerate them into their sensitive form. The bleaching process takes place within one minute, so adaptation to bright light is quick. But regeneration is slow: The eye needs about 10 minutes to adapt to a drop from the bright illumination of a reading lamp to that of nighttime highway lighting. Complete adaptation requires more than 10 hours—but then the average eye can detect light $1/100,000$ as bright as when it is accustomed to full sunlight.

Modern eye medicines are compounded with ingredients that do indeed, in the words of the advertisements, "get the red out." They contain decongestants, which shrink blood vessels to reduce inflammation. However, their effects are short-lived, and under continued irritation the blood vessels soon dilate again. After repeated use of the eye drops, an effect known as rebound may make the vessels dilate even in the absence of irritation.

The drugs in eye drops also bring side effects. They sometimes cause allergic reactions, such as rashes or breathing difficulties, and they may interact with other eye medicines, such as the cleaning and lubricating agents used with contact lenses, to irritate the eye. For one small group of patients, sufferers from a relatively rare form of the major eye disease glaucoma *(page 92)*, eye drops containing decongestants bring a special hazard. They dilate the pupil of the eye, and pupil dilation can trigger a severe glaucoma attack.

Not all eye drops contain decongestants. Some are simply artificial tears: a salty solution that more or less duplicates the chemical composition of real tears, sometimes thickened with the innocuous compound methylcellulose. They assist natural tears to spread a long-lasting film over the eyeball, and can be useful for persons who are chronically deficient in tear production—victims of arthritis, for example—and for those who occasionally suffer tired eyes.

If you use eye drops of any kind, follow a few simple rules based on a need for absolute cleanliness. Eye preparations must, by law, be sterile when they are shipped from the pharmaceutical plant, but when the bottles are unsealed and their contents transferred to an eyecup or a dropper, these solutions can become transmitters of disease. Eyecups are more hazardous, "an outmoded and dangerous method of delivering eye medication," said Dr. David Miller of Harvard. They are difficult to sterilize and can cause injury to the eye. The ideal dispenser, in the opinion of most physicians, is a squeeze bottle, which helps avoid the contamination often introduced when a dropper is set down on a countertop or table.

Giving eyes a workout to sharpen skills

Good eyesight means more than 20/20 vision: It encompasses a wide range of reflexes that give scope and flexibility to vision and coordinate signals to and from the brain. The exercises pictured here help sharpen the abilities involved—just as practicing a musical composition improves performance. But such vision therapy is controversial. Although exercises can enhance such everyday skills as hitting a tennis ball, doctors point out that, despite the claims of enthusiasts, they do not change sight—only the capacity to use it. No exercise can substitute for glasses or surgery.

HONING THE SENSE OF PERIPHERAL VISION
In an unfamiliar room, point your eyes at one object and see how many other objects you can identify without moving your head and eyes. Then try the same exercise while walking down a street. Skill in using peripheral vision—seeing "out of the corner of the eye"—helps automobile drivers spot dangers at the side.

USING EYES TOGETHER TO SEE A FUSED IMAGE
Place two index cards, one marked with a circle and the other with a square, on adjoining walls at eye level, three feet from the corner. Facing the circle, angle a mirror in front of your nose to reflect the square, adjusting it until you see the circle inside the square. This sort of visual teamwork is vital to depth perception.

Before using a squeeze bottle or a dropper, wash your hands thoroughly. Then, watching yourself in a mirror, pull a lower eyelid down with the fleshy tip—not the nail—of one finger. Hold the bottle or dropper in the other hand, and squeeze out drops so that they fall into the small pouch you have made in the eyelid; take special care not to touch any part of the eye, including the lashes, with the end of the nozzle or dropper. If you are using a dropper, put it back in the bottle immediately; do not set it down on a countertop. Finally, blink a few times to spread the medicine, then keep your eye closed for a few minutes to increase the absorption of the liquid.

Inaccessible to drops or washes, but more disturbing to look at than a bloodshot eye, is a bright red spot in the clear white of an eyeball. It is exactly what it looks like—blood, in this case hemorrhaging from a vessel on the surface of the eyeball but within the enveloping protective film of the conjunctiva. Typically it occurs for no discernible reason. However, it can result from an injury. Even a bout of severe

sneezing, coughing or vomiting, or extreme physical exertion, such as heavy lifting or the labor of childbirth, can trigger a rise in blood pressure and a tiny blowout in a blood vessel. The white of the eye is suffused with blood, not necessarily at the moment of exertion but perhaps hours later, when the triggering event is long forgotten.

Such bleeding is almost always painless and harmless; you need to consult a physician only when it dims vision, occurs repeatedly or follows a physical injury. Otherwise, the best treatment is simply time. Depending upon the size of the bloody area and the body's natural healing properties, the spilled blood will be reabsorbed in one to three weeks; recovery can be slightly speeded by warm compresses, applied to the affected eye the second day and several times a day thereafter. Vision is virtually unaffected during the waiting period, and if the spectacular appearance of the eye is bothersome, ordinary sunglasses will hide the redness.

Red eyes can be symptoms of more than fatigue or harmless bleeding, however. They also arise from allergies,

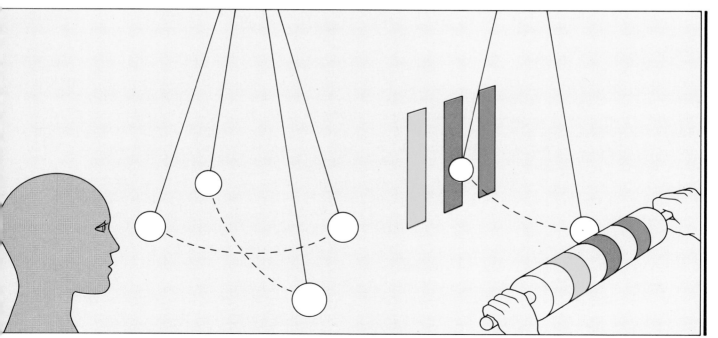

LEARNING TO KEEP YOUR EYE ON THE BALL
Vision pursuit—the skill used in catching an airborne Frisbee—may be sharpened with the aid of a ball suspended from the ceiling at eye level. Swing the ball from side to side, then back and forth, following it with your eyes. The eyes practice moving and focusing rapidly and smoothly in this exercise.

COORDINATING EYES AND BODY
Wind stripes of three colors on a rolling pin, then put strips on a wall in the same color pattern. Suspend a ball from the ceiling at eye level, two feet from the wall, and bounce the ball against the wall strips with the matching stripe on the rolling pin. This improves the coordination of visual signals and body movement.

chemical irritation and several kinds of infections. Such inflammations often bring an uncomfortable sensitivity to light and may cause the eye to run, swell up and even stick shut. If they persist they can cause serious harm or may be a sign of dangerous disease; any eye ailment that does not begin to go away after several days should be brought to a physician's attention.

Causes and cures of inflammation

The most common of these inflammations is conjunctivitis, which affects the white of the eye. If the infection is caused by bacteria—as it is in the "pinkeye" that so frequently plagues young school children—its elimination can be hastened by a doctor's prescription for antibiotic ointment or drops. Conjunctivitis spreads easily among family members. The hand that rubs inflamed eyelids is a common transmitter. To avoid contagion, the patient should remain at home and wash his hands frequently, using his own washcloth and towel. The discharge should be removed several times a day with a fresh gauze pad dipped in warm water. An eye patch should not be worn because it harbors the discharge, creating a breeding ground for more bacteria, but dark glasses ease the eyes.

Conjunctivitis is often caused by a virus and accompanies a viral disease such as the common cold or influenza. In such cases, medicines will not help because viruses are generally invulnerable to antibiotics. Viral conjunctivitis can be distinguished from the bacterial type by symptoms: The viral eye infection produces relatively little thick discharge, but copious tearing, and it is often accompanied by sore throat and fever and by swelling of the eye's drainage glands, located just in front of the ears.

Allergic conjunctivitis is brought on by the pollen, feathers, animal hairs, foods, drugs or cosmetics that cause hay fever-like symptoms and asthma. Its special signs include swollen eyelids, severe itching, a minimal, stringy discharge and moderate tearing. In allergic conjunctivitis that is linked to the seasons, antihistamines may help; so, too, may cold compresses or ice packs applied to the eye, and an air conditioner in the bedroom.

Among the common allergy triggers are cosmetics, which have turned out to be double and even triple threats. They cause allergic reactions in some people, and they can produce chemical irritation or transmit infection as well. An opened container of oily cosmetics provides an excellent culture medium for disease organisms; if the cosmetics are passed from one person to another, they can carry infection to every eye they touch. The danger is greatest, perhaps, among adolescent girls, who often share their latest discoveries in brands of make-up. The American Pharmaceutical Association's *Handbook of Nonprescription Drugs* reported that at one high school in California the contents of a single container of eye make-up had spread bacterial conjunctivitis to no fewer than 75 girls.

The third threat of cosmetics arises from chemical irritation. The cure is simple: Wash away the offending material. Most chemical conjunctivitis, however, is caused by more pervasive and longer-lasting substances: chlorine in swimming pools, salt in sea water, fertilizers, pesticides, soaps, antiseptics, cigarette smoke and air pollutants. Artificial tears can briefly supplement natural healing, and swimmers can wear goggles to protect themselves against chlorine or salt water, but a smog alert may make it impossible to escape eye inflammation.

Bacteria not only infect the white of the eye to cause conjunctivitis but also attack various parts of the eyelid: the edge near the eyelashes, glands near the lashes or glands just inside the lid. Like conjunctivitis, eyelid inflammations require a doctor's treatment only if they are painful or if they do not improve after a few days of home treatment.

Sties, the familiar tender red bumps that pop out on the edge of a lid, can usually be treated with hot compresses applied for 15 minutes, three or four times a day. Never squeeze a sty, but always wipe away any pus that seeps out of it; the pus can spread infection. If you suffer constantly recurring sties, consult a physician, for they are sometimes an early sign of diabetes.

Similar to a sty but slower to develop and resolve is the chalazion, a cyst that forms when a gland inside a lid becomes plugged. Sometimes infection is the cause, but often the only symptom is a painless, persistent lump. Eventually, the gland becomes distended, hard (the Latin name of the cyst means "hailstone") and more or less permanent. Warm compresses generally will make the lump disappear in a week or so.

Blepharitis ("eyelid inflammation") is an infection that seldom goes away without aid from a doctor. It commonly attacks adolescents and is characterized by red-rimmed, swollen eyelids, severe itching, and a fine crusting and scaling of the skin at the base of the eyelashes. Blepharitis usually occurs together with abnormally increased dandruff that contains some infectious bacteria, and this situation calls for treatment on two fronts: frequent scalp shampoos to prevent the bacteria from spreading, and prescription eye drops to cure the infection.

Although ordinary eye ailments are generally harmless, eye injuries, which are almost as common, are not. Every year some 40,000 Americans severely damage one or both of their eyes in accidents, and about 1,500 of them lose their sight. Even a black eye, the subject of so many jokes, is nothing to laugh about.

Although the eye is protected by its location, recessed in a socket that is surrounded by the armor of skull and cheekbone, a blow to that part of the face can cause a hemorrhage, a cataract, a dislocated lens or a detached retina *(pages 128-129)*. The symptoms of such severe damage will usually show up almost immediately as double vision, blurred vision or increasing pain, but not always. Any time an eye suffers a direct hit, the best rule is to see a physician even in the absence of symptoms.

Ordinarily a blow is absorbed by the surrounding armor, and the injury is limited to the skin and the tiny blood vessels beneath it, leaving nothing more serious than the characteristic black-and-blue bruise mark around the eye. The treatment for a simple black eye begins with an ice pack or cold compress (a compress is almost as effective as an ice pack and a good deal more comfortable) applied for 15 minutes at one-hour intervals for four or five hours. After each application, check again for any signs of blurriness or pain. Next day you will find that the swelling has gone down, but you may also find that the skin around your eye—now a genuine shiner—has deepened in color. Switch to warm compresses, applied frequently, to speed the absorption of the hemorrhaged blood. One old remedy that is not worth trying is a bloody sirloin steak against the eye; it has no value beyond enriching the butcher.

Why everybody needs safety goggles

Walking into a door is not likely to do any lasting damage to sight. A much greater threat is presented when flying objects, chemicals or radiation strike the eye itself. Injuries sustained then are serious. They can almost always be prevented by goggles, which are a safeguard needed far more often than most people recognize.

Safety goggles, which can be bought inexpensively at hardware stores, are not only essential in factories but are recommended by doctors for many sports, for most repair jobs at home and for many gardening and cleaning chores. They are needed for any work that calls for power tools—and eye experts insist they should be worn for such simple jobs as chipping stone or hammering nails. They are a wise precaution for anyone playing a sport involving very fast-moving balls, such as squash and racquetball, and on the open road they provide joggers and cyclists with the only practical shield against the pebbles and grit thrown into the air by speeding cars.

Because chemical burns can be as devastating as any blow or cut, wearing goggles is a wise precaution whenever you use such chemicals as oven cleaners, paint removers, powerful detergents, pesticides and varnishes. Goggles are eye-saving necessities in all work with plaster and lime, which contain corrosive alkalies, and they should be worn by anyone doing any work beneath the hood of an automobile, especially near the battery.

Special goggles, tinted dark, are needed to guard eyes against an insidious danger from light—not the light of a lamp, which is harmless, but the invisible ultraviolet light emitted by the sun, sunlamps and arc-welding equipment such as is often used for auto repair. Ultraviolet light burns the outer protective layer of the eyeball and can quickly lead to what is called snow blindness (it often is caused by sunlight reflected from snow). The effect is not noticed until six to nine hours after exposure, when the eyes feel as though full of sand and become painfully sensitive to light, and vision dims and blurs. According to a definitive text, ''If the damage has been deep enough to cause sloughing of the corneal tissue, the eye is almost certainly lost.'' Such harm is uncommon. More often, rest in a darkened room brings full recovery in a few days.

Because of the risk of ultraviolet burn, skiers should always wear tinted goggles. Ultraviolet radiation is stronger in the mountains, and snow reflects it up from below, so that eyebrows, lashes and lids cannot block it out. Sidewalk superintendents who watch welders should look away as soon as the work begins. And anyone who insists on cultivating a suntan should protect his eyes with opaque eye ''occluders,'' which block all light rays. (However, neither natural nor artificial suntan is recommended by medical authorities because it can lead to skin cancer.)

Far more serious—and also, happily, far more rare—than an ordinary ultraviolet-light burn is the effect of gazing directly at the sun. Normally, the sun's rays are so intense that few people are tempted to do this. At the beginning and end of an eclipse, however, the light is reduced and curiosity impels people to look up at the sun. As far back as the Fifth Century B.C., Socrates warned people against the practice. The reason is simple: The eye focuses the sun's rays on the most sensitive part of the retina, and these rays can burn it exactly as a magnifying glass burns a dry leaf. Sunglasses, darkened photographic film and that old standby, smoked glass, are little or no protection. The safest way to see an eclipse is on televison.

When to take an eye exam—and from whom

In spite of all precautions, eye accidents will occur, and their victims must be healed. Disease threatens or attacks the eye, with consequences that range from discomfort to blindness, and it must be averted or cured. And sooner or later, most people need eyeglasses. The need generally begins during childhood or adolescence and changes throughout life, so that the eyes require new lens prescriptions from time to time. Oddly enough, many people who should be using eyeglasses are not aware of it, for the eye has amazing power to adapt to abnormalities.

Dr. David Miller of Harvard recently related the case of a nurse who worked with him in surgery. While she was preparing the instrument table for an operation, he wrote, ''One of the very fine sutures, with the needle attached, fell onto the black-and-white checkered floor by accident. As I walked into the room, she was on her hands and knees looking for the suture and needle. How futile, I thought, to look for something so fine on such a confusing background. All at once she stopped, reached down, and came up grinning with the suture. 'What amazing eyesight!' I exclaimed. Not long after this episode, she came into the eye clinic for a routine checkup,'' Dr. Miller wrote, and proved to be extremely nearsighted. Yet, he noted, ''Under my very eyes, this nurse had performed a visual miracle.''

The scheduling of eye checkups is important. Most doctors now recommend that the first complete examination take place when a child is about three years old; vision is rapidly stabilizing at that stage, but it is still flexible enough to be corrected for problems of development. For children with healthy eyes, the second visit should be made at the age of five or six, just before they start elementary school. From then on, those youngsters who wear corrective lenses should be examined every 18 months or so; those who do not, at intervals of two or three years.

Even more important than the schedule of examinations, of course, is the choice of examiner. There are three kinds of professionals specializing in eye care, and the differences among them confuse many people. An ophthalmologist is a medical doctor with advanced training in eye disorders; this specialist tests eyes for all kinds of diseases and defects, prescribes corrective lenses, administers eye medicines and performs eye operations.

An optometrist is not a physician but rather an expert in testing eyes for focusing defects and in prescribing lenses to correct them. This practitioner does not treat other disorders, but may detect them in the course of an examination and will

Mysterious machines that probe the eye

Even a routine eye examination requires an array of machines that seem suited to a science-fiction movie. Their magnifying lenses, high-intensity light beams and delicate probes enable a doctor to watch the eye in action, look for signs of disease or optical flaws and even measure pressure inside the eyeball.

A typical examination begins with preliminary tests for muscle balance, depth perception, peripheral vision, color blindness *(see page 76)* and faulty focus. Most involve such simple maneuvers as reading an eye chart with one eye covered, looking at pictures through 3-D glasses, and following a penlight or the doctor's moving finger with the eyes. But next the doctor studies the interior of the eye, taking advantage of the fact that when the pupil is enlarged and kept open with dilating drops, it becomes a two-way window. For some tests, he may put in additional drops that paralyze the focusing muscles (and cause temporary blurring). Using the instruments pictured below and on the following pages, the doctor can examine the inner structures of the organ in detail, measure the exact angle of error that results when light rays are bounced off a misshapen eye, and prescribe corrective lenses to bring vision into proper focus.

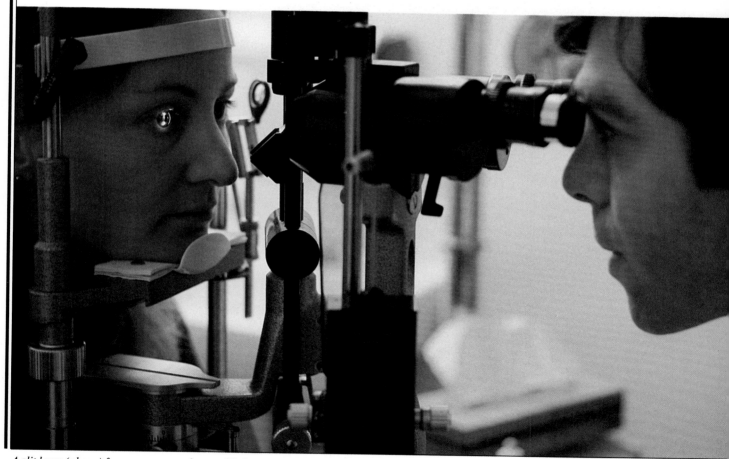

A slit lamp (above) focuses a narrow beam of light at a sharp angle into a patient's eye while the doctor inspects inner and outer sections of her eye through a microscope. The light reaching the eye at an angle reveals defects not visible under head-on illumination—just as an apparently clear watch crystal will show scratches in light that angles across it.

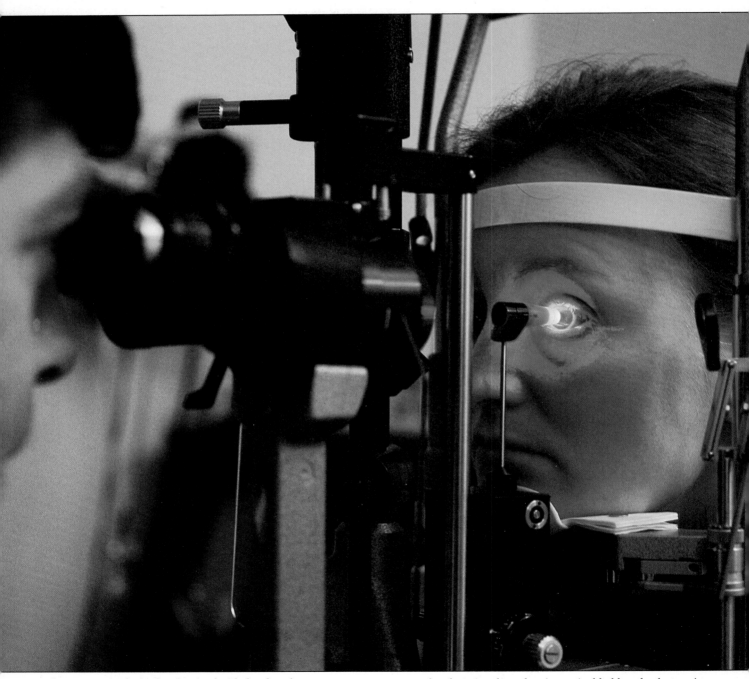

On an eye anesthetized and stained with dye that glows
phosphorescent blue, the doctor tests for glaucoma—excessive
pressure from internal fluids—with an applanation tonometer.
The device measures internal pressure by indicating the force
needed to flatten a circular area on the cornea with a plastic rod,
visible above as a bright blue next to the patient's eye. While
gently advancing the rod on its vertical holder, the doctor views
the eye through a prism that works like the rangefinder on a
camera. Dye on the surface of the eyeball, forming a bead around
the rod, appears as a split image through the prism. When the
cornea is flat, the split images will line up, and the force required
for flattening is indicated on a scale (not visible).

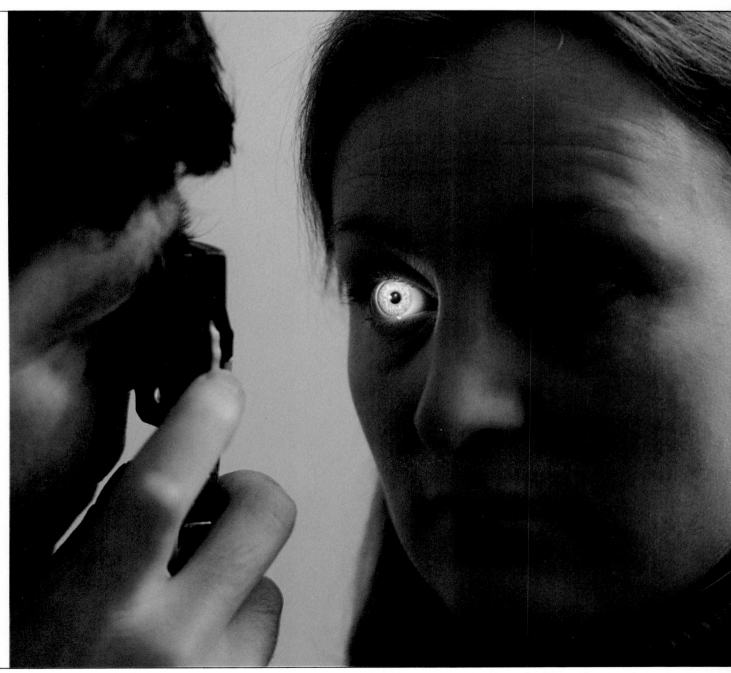

After the patient's pupils have been dilated and her near-focusing muscles temporarily paralyzed with eye drops, the doctor asks her to look across the darkened room while he surveys the rear wall of her inner eye through an ophthalmoscope. A light in the instrument's shaft bounces off an angled mirror just above it into the eye and onto the retina; from a series of lenses on a rotating wheel under his finger, the doctor selects one that gives him a clear view. Because the retina is the only part of the body where nerves and blood vessels are visible, the doctor making an ophthalmoscope examination can detect signs of disorders such as high blood pressure and diabetes as well as damage to the retina and optic nerve.

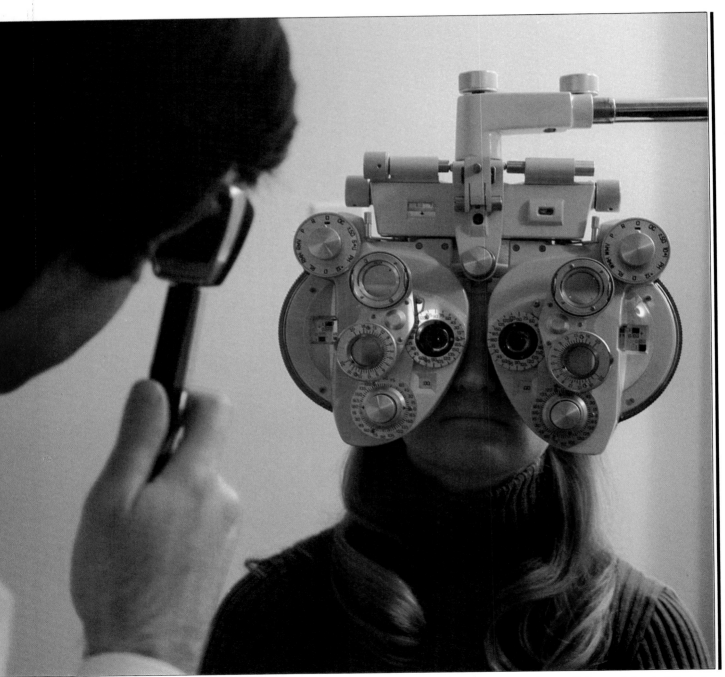

While the patient looks at an eye chart, the doctor checks her focusing accuracy with a hand-held retinoscope and the adjustable lenses of the refractor in front of her face. A mirror in the retinoscope directs a light beam through the refractor into the patient's pupil; if the eye focuses properly, the pupil fills completely with a reflected red glow. If the patient is nearsighted or farsighted, the red glow forms a light streak that is deflected right or left by the improper focus. After using the retinoscope to estimate the degree of focusing error, the doctor then confirms his findings and determines the prescription for eyeglasses by trying various lenses on the refractor until he finds the combination that lets the patient see the chart most clearly.

refer those cases to an ophthalmologist. However, an optometrist sells and fits lenses, a service that only a few ophthalmologists provide.

The optician is a licensed technician comparable to a pharmacist. This specialist fills prescriptions for lenses and fits eyeglasses and, in some places, contact lenses to the customer; an optician performs no examinations and prescribes no remedies.

The obvious choice for all-round eye care and regular examinations is the most versatile of these professionals, the ophthalmologist physician. However, when corrective lenses are known to be the only requirement, the more narrowly trained optometrist is sometimes the more skilled; after all, fitting lenses is his only work.

An ophthalmologist's full examination is an exhaustive affair, lasting up to an hour and requiring a number of strange-looking instruments *(pages 71-74)*. It begins with a medical history and a scrutiny of the external parts of the eyes—the lids and visible part of the eyeball—for signs of redness, inflammation or growths. The doctor may check blinking and tearing reflexes, using tiny lengths of absorbent paper to soak up tears from the area behind the lower lids. Next is a check of the pressure of the fluid within the eye, a clue to the presence of glaucoma.

The ophthalmologist then goes on to study the internal parts of the eye, aided by the unique anatomy of the organ. Alone among the structures of the body, the eye contains transparent components: the cornea, the open pupil and the lens behind it, and the fluids that fill the eyeball. Without X-rays or incisions, an ophthalmologist can examine the interior of the eye.

But mainly the examiner investigates the performance of the eyes in various acts of seeing. One test checks color vision *(page 76),* another eye-muscle coordination, impairment of which causes cross-eyes or walleyes *(pages 115-118)*. One critical test deals with peripheral vision—the ability to see to the left or right and up or down without moving the head or eyeballs. In a typical test of this aspect of vision, the patient is instructed to close one eye and to fix the other on the eye or nose of the examiner; then, slowly, the examiner moves a pen or a finger from each of four diagonal directions toward the line of sight. The patient reports the moment at which the pen or finger can be detected; a failure to spot the object until it nearly reaches the line of sight is an indication of abnormality—and of the need for further testing to detect the possible presence of glaucoma, a detached retina or some other serious affliction.

What the charts tell

Tests for peripheral or color vision have consequences for only a minority of those who take them; not many people, after all, suffer from glaucoma or color blindness. Evaluations of visual acuity, on the other hand, affect almost everyone. It is these examinations that determine whether a patient needs glasses, and if so, what kind of glasses.

The standard test, which measures the ability to make out details of distant objects, is familiar enough. With one eye covered, the patient reads aloud the lines of letters or numbers on a chart or projection screen 20 feet away. Each line is set in a type size smaller than the one above it; when the subject reaches a line whose individual characters are too small to be distinguished, the test for that eye comes to an end and the other eye is tested. The smallest type that the patient is able to read gives a numerical grade for vision—20/100, 20/40 or the 20/20 that is generally considered normal. Each eye receives its own rating—a person may have 20/20 vision in one eye and 20/40 in the other.

The ratings compare a patient's eyes with those of an anonymous young man who lived more than a century ago in the Netherlands. The eye chart is called the Snellen chart, after the Dutch ophthalmologist, Dr. Herman Snellen, who perfected it in 1864. Having worked out a system of printed lines graduated in size, Dr. Snellen sought for a standard or bench mark against which to measure the sight of his subjects. He found it in his own assistant, a man of acute and exceptionally consistent eyesight, which was arbitrarily adopted by Dr. Snellen as normal. The name of the assistant is lost to history, but people all over the world have been pitting their sight against his ever since.

The first number in a Snellen rating is the distance of the

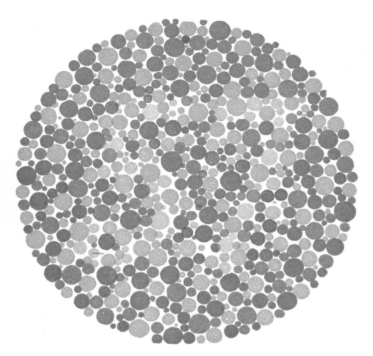

To a color-blind person, the picture above might be only an array of colored dots, its number 57 indiscernible. This color pattern is one of a series, each containing a number visible to people with normal color perception. Failure to pick out the 57 would not, by itself, confirm color blindness; several similar patterns are needed to complete the test.

subject from the chart—always 20 feet. The second number, which is different for each line on the chart, is the distance at which Dr. Snellen's assistant was able to read that line.

One of the smaller sizes of type on a Snellen chart fills the 20/20 line; a person who can read that far down, and no farther, has 20/20 vision, because at 20 feet from the chart he can read exactly what Dr. Snellen's assistant could read at the same distance. Farther up the chart, in larger type, is the 20/40 line; the patient who cannot read below it sees clearly at 20 feet what a person with normal vision can see at 40. (This patient could benefit from glasses, but 20/40 vision in either eye is sufficient qualification for a driver's license in most places.)

The very top of the chart is generally a single enormous *E,* the 20/200 line, indicating the level of legal blindness, its type so large that a person of normal sight can read it 200 feet away. But the chart also contains lines for the unusually sharp-eyed, those people who could beat Dr. Snellen's assistant in the test. Down at the bottom, in type that to most people looks like flyspecks, are 20/15 and 20/10 lines, which the assistant could not read without advancing to positions only 15 or 10 feet from the chart.

Near vision nowadays is tested in much the same way, usually with cards bearing printed paragraphs in graduated type sizes. The cards are held exactly 14 inches from the eyes of the patient—because 14 inches was chosen as the typical distance for reading printed matter. Thus, a rating of 14/14 represents normal near vision; 14/21, 14/28 and 14/35 stand for progressively greater degrees of near-vision impairment.

Using lenses for clear vision

The tests grade the eyes' ability to focus without glasses. The goal is generally prescriptions for lenses that will correct distance vision to 20/20 and near vision to 14/14. These lenses quite literally correct refractive error, altering the paths of light rays to cancel out the misfocusing introduced by defects in the eye's own focusing system.

The eye does not focus the way a camera does. Most of the job is done by the cornea, which is not adjustable. The lens, behind the cornea, is adjustable to make the slight changes necessary to focus on the retina, at the back of the eyeball, the rays coming from near objects or from distant ones. Unlike a camera lens, the human lens does not move forward and back to make these focus adjustments; it changes its shape. Surrounding muscles tighten to slacken ligaments and allow the lens to bulge into a convex shape for close-up viewing, or they relax to let the ligaments pull the lens into the thinner shape needed for distance viewing.

Variations in any part of this system—the shape of the cornea, the activity of muscles and, most important, the distance from cornea to retina—affect the ability to focus and may make glasses necessary. These variations introduce three common defects of vision: farsightedness (called hyperopia by doctors), nearsightedness (myopia) and astigmatism *(pages 82-83)*.

Farsightedness is caused by an eyeball that is slightly shorter front to back than a normal eye, or by a cornea and lens that together have less light-bending power than average, or by a combination of these causes. These conditions may have little effect on the ability to see objects 20 feet or more away, particularly in young people, because light rays from distant objects are essentially parallel and require little bending inward to make them converge at a point on the retina. The strength of youthful focusing muscles can easily adjust the lens to provide the small amount of bending required. However, near objects—a printed page, for example—do appear blurred, because the rays of light are diverging when they reach the eye; with a retina unusually close to the cornea and lens, or a cornea and lens that are weak in bending power, even strong focusing muscles may not be able to bend these diverging rays to bring them together at a point within the space available inside the eyeball.

Nearly everyone is born with some degree of farsightedness, but the condition usually corrects itself as a child grows. When it does not, minor farsightedness may not be noticed for years unless the youngster undergoes periodic eye examinations—and even then, an ophthalmologist may not prescribe corrective lenses if the child has no symptoms of eyestrain. As an adult comes to depend increasingly on his eyes for close work and as his power to control his eyes'

lenses diminishes, even mild farsightedness begins to cause blurring. The remedy is simple and effective: The refractive error can be corrected by an external convex lens that adds its own refractive power to that of the eye's and delivers a precisely focused image on the retina.

Nearsightedness, or myopia, a condition in which near objects are seen more clearly than distant ones, is caused by defects exactly opposite to those introducing farsightedness: The eyeball is slightly too long, front to back, to match the focusing power of the cornea and lens. The light rays that they refract come to a focus at a point somewhere in front of the retina, then diverge; at the retina, the diverging rays produce a blurred image. A concave corrective lens spreads the rays before they reach the eye, so that the final focus at the retina is precise.

Few babies are born nearsighted; the condition generally reveals its existence after the third birthday. Typical giveaways are squinting, sitting very close to a television screen, learning difficulties at school and poor performance in sports. At puberty the development of nearsightedness accelerates, and some adolescents need new lens prescriptions every six months or so.

The rapid development of this defect during the years of formal schooling has revived an old controversy. For years parents and grandparents have insisted that too much reading makes young people nearsighted; for years ophthalmologists have insisted that nearsightedness stems from an innate anatomical problem. The experts may have been wrong. In 1970, for example, Francis A. Young of Washington State University checked the eyesight of the inhabitants of the village of Nuvuk in Point Barrow, Alaska, an isolated community of people of Eskimo ancestry. He found that parents and grandparents, who were generally illiterate, had almost no nearsightedness, while among the villagers less than 25 years old, who all had been taught to read, about 60 per cent suffered from this impairment.

No less striking are the results of earlier research by a number of scientists in the United States and Canada. Among grade-school students, 10 per cent were nearsighted; among high-school students, 20 per cent; among undergraduate college students, 40 per cent; and among graduate students, 50 per cent, a proportion far greater than among people of the same age who do not attend graduate school. In the light of such evidence, ophthalmologists have been modifying their position. Harvard's Dr. Miller recently suggested that although nearsightedness is probably hereditary, it is most likely to reveal itself "if the subject reads a great deal during his teens and twenties."

Astigmatism, the third kind of refractive error, distorts or blurs images at all distances, and may be combined with farsightedness or nearsightedness. The basic problem lies in a cornea that, rather than being symmetrical and smooth, is rough or misshapen. The cornea can distort vertical, horizontal or diagonal lines; if its entire surface is irregular or bumpy, the eye will not focus on any object. If the distortion has the effect of tilting the field of vision, a victim may tilt his head slightly to the opposite side to compensate. A special lens with a slight cylindrical bulge corrects the distortion.

Eventually another visual defect impairs the vision of most people: presbyopia, a symptom of aging (the term is derived from the Greek words for "old sight"). In the mid-40s the eye's ability to focus upon close work begins to fail because the lens becomes progressively harder, less flexible and thus more difficult to focus.

The simplest correction for presbyopia is a pair of so-called reading glasses, with convex lenses designed to help the eye focus on objects 14 inches away. But most people add presbyopia to an existing vision problem and need two kinds of lenses, generally combined into bifocal glasses, which correct presbyopia at the bottom and the earlier error at the top. Bifocals can prove awkward—switching the eyes from one part of the lens to the other can be tricky, and descending a flight of stairs or stepping off a curb can at first be downright dangerous; the inconvenient alternative of two pairs of glasses may be preferable.

Getting the right glasses

You can buy inexpensive reading glasses in the dime store in many places, simply trying on spectacles from the counter tray until you find a pair that brings a printed page into sharp focus. This is not recommended; eyeglasses should be custom-made to the individual prescription by a qualified technician. Yet the qualifications of the dispensers of eyeglasses are regulated in fewer than half the states in the United States (by contrast, pharmacists throughout the country must be licensed). One guide to the expertise of an eyeglass dealer is a plaque in the office or shop indicating that the seller meets standards established by one of the professional associations, such as the American Board of Opticians, the National Contact Lens Examiners or the Guild of Prescription Opticians of America.

Even the qualified dispensers generally do not fill the prescriptions themselves; most order the specified lenses from optical laboratories that specialize in grinding eyeglass lenses. And the quality of the laboratories' work has been called into question. A 1977 report revealed that optometrists had had to reject from 5 per cent to as many as 25 per cent of the lenses they ordered. To protect yourself against incorrectly ground lenses, do not accept a new pair of glasses until the seller has checked them against your prescription on an optical testing machine.

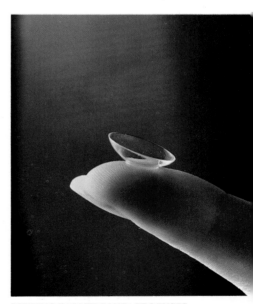

PUTTING IN SOFT CONTACT LENSES
With clean hands, stand in front of a mirror and place the lens, wet with solution and edges up, on your index finger.

Modern eyeglass lenses are made of either plastic or shatter-resistant glass. Plastic costs slightly more, yet most people prefer it. Plastic lenses are lighter, and therefore especially suitable for thick lenses and for the outsized styles that sometimes are in fashion; they are also less likely to fog over with moisture. On the other hand, plastic lenses scratch more easily than glass, even with the antiscratch coating often used now, and the scratches, however superficial, cannot be polished away.

Many people choose tinted lenses. Aside from a stylish look and a small degree of additional comfort for some light-sensitive people, the choice offers no medical benefit—and the selection of a tint should always be made carefully. Pale tints will not diminish your color perception or reduce your vision; darker ones will, however, and they should be worn only in bright sunlight.

The frame you choose from the hundreds of models available is mainly, but not entirely, a matter of personal taste. If you do strenuous physical work or engage in active sports, you will be better off with plastic frames than with rimless or wire models, which more easily bend out of alignment. A frame should be both comfortable and snug at the ears and nose; one that slides down to the tip of the nose distorts vision. A certain amount of inevitable distortion occurs at the outer margins of a lens—and the bigger the lens, the greater the distortion. Finally, remember that the optician will offer you frames that are empty of lenses; if you cannot see well without glasses, consider bringing a friend to judge your appearance.

Once purchased, eyeglasses must be kept clean, reasonably scratch-free, and properly seated on the face. The American Optometric Association has drawn up a set of rules for eyeglass care:

● Clean lenses twice a day, either with warm water and soap or with a commercial eyeglass-cleansing solution, using the pads of your fingers to loosen any spots or smudges; dry the lenses with a tissue or with a soft, clean cloth. When necessary, scrub the nose pads, bridge and hinges with a toothbrush. Exercise special care when handling plastic lenses. Do not clean them with silicone tissues, and never wipe them while they are dry.

● When you are not wearing your glasses, store them in a

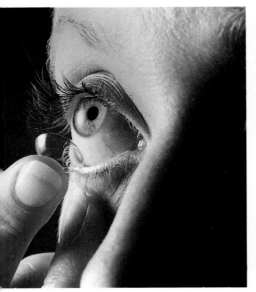

With the middle finger of your other hand, hold down the lower eyelid and stare upward. Bring the lens close to the white of the eye, just below the cornea.

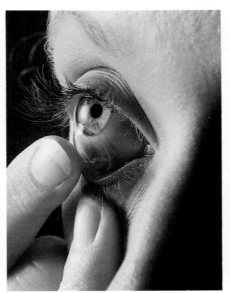

Without blinking, place the lens on the white of the eye, pressing gently to squeeze out air trapped underneath the lens and to smooth out any wrinkles in the lens.

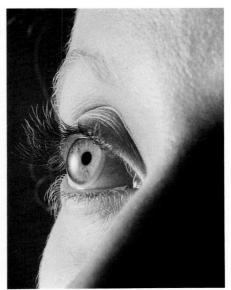

Remove your fingers and look down— the lens will center itself. Hard contacts are inserted similarly, but placed over the pupil while looking straight ahead.

case; hinged cases are better than slip-in cases for plastic lenses because they inflict fewer scratches. If the glasses will be off only for a short time, lay them down folded, with the lenses facing upward, so that the lenses do not touch any surface.

● Whenever you put on or remove your glasses, use both hands, holding the temples at about their midpoints and sliding the frames onto or off your head; using one hand will eventually bend the frame or weaken its joints, and thus misalign the lenses.

● Have your optician readjust your frames every once in a while. Sooner or later all frames loosen or get out of line, altering the alignment of their lenses and impairing the correction of your vision; rimless and wire frames are the most vulnerable.

Pros and cons of contact lenses

Although most people wear eyeglasses in frames, the popularity of contact lenses—disks that float on the eyeball—is growing rapidly. Leonardo da Vinci developed a design for contact lenses in 1508, and as far back as 1888, scientists working independently of each other in Switzerland and France made glass contacts. But not until good transparent plastic became available in the 1930s did contact lenses become practical. By the mid-1960s about four million Americans (including President Lyndon B. Johnson) were wearing them, and by 1977 the number had grown to 14 million. Even chickens have been fitted with contact lenses. Red-tinted, the fowl lenses prolong chickens' lives by making blood invisible to them; the sight of blood can stimulate chickens to peck at one another in disastrous battles for supremacy that may kill off a quarter of a flock.

The name "contact" is somewhat misleading: Smaller and thinner than the nail of the little finger, the lens does not actually touch the eyeball; rather, it floats upon a microscopically thin cushion of tears. It adheres to the tear layer wherever it is placed, and thus it follows the movements of the eyeball, maintaining a position directly in front of the cornea, so that the wearer views all objects through the distortion-free center of the lens. Eyeglasses distort vision whenever the wearer happens to glance to one side, or up or down.

Two main kinds of contact lenses are available. The older, "hard" lenses, made of a stiff plastic, are the most durable. Many people have difficulty in adapting to them because the eyes initially attempt to reject the inflexible disks. New wearers may need four weeks or more to adjust to wearing them all day.

Hard contacts must be removed each night because they become uncomfortable after 12 to 14 hours and they block transmission of the oxygen needed by the cornea. They should be worn every day: If the wearer substitutes glasses for a couple of days, the eyes must then readapt to the contact lenses. Specialized pharmaceutical products must be used with hard contacts daily to ensure comfort and cleanliness. Among these are a wetting solution, which helps the water-resistant plastic pick up a uniform film of tears; a soaking solution, in which lenses are stored overnight; and cleaning solutions, which eliminate oily eye secretions that soaking solutions may not remove.

The newer soft lenses, which have the consistency of gelatin, are made of a plastic that retains its flexibility by absorbing moisture from the eye. They conform readily to the contours of the cornea; therefore, wearers adapt to them quickly, seldom experience irritation and can keep them on during active sports. Their greatest advantage, perhaps, is their versatility. Soft-lens wearers can keep them on for as long as 18 hours, or they can switch to ordinary glasses for days at a time without going through the stress of readaptation when the contacts are reinserted. However, soft lenses must be cleaned and sterilized with special solutions, according to precise schedules and procedures. Soft contacts are more expensive than hard lenses, do not last as long and cannot be given the complex shapes needed to correct some defects, such as astigmatism.

New types called extended-wear lenses are, unlike others, permeable to oxygen. They have been worn as long as four weeks at a time by some patients.

Fitting a contact lens requires a skillful doctor and a cooperative patient, particularly during the adjustment period. As many as six visits may be needed to get a satisfactory fit;

frequent follow-up visits in the first weeks and semiannual checkups make the fitting process far more expensive than that for corrective glasses. Even among those who get an expert fit, about 30 per cent fail to make a satisfactory adaptation to hard lenses; the failure figure for soft-lens wearers is about 10 per cent.

Although each type of contact lens calls for specific precautions and requirements, some basic rules apply to all:

● Never wear a lens that is nicked or chipped; it can damage the cornea.

● Insert lenses in a clean, dust-free room, and be sure your hands are clean.

● Use the wetting agent recommended for your lenses before inserting them; never use saliva, which creates a risk of bacterial infection.

● Take care to place each lens in the appropriate eye; switches caused by carelessness in storage or handling can produce eyestrain and blurring of vision.

● If you use eye make-up, insert the lenses first, then apply the cosmetics sparingly. Avoid oily products, which can smear, and the adhesives used with false eyelashes, which can flake off.

● When using hair spray or deodorant spray, keep your eyes closed until the air has cleared. Keep them closed, too, under a hair dryer; the heat can evaporate tears and leave the lenses in direct contact with the corneas, where they can cause abrasion.

● Remove contact lenses when swimming; they can easily be washed out of the eyes.

Contact-lens wearers must be alert to the signs of corneal abrasion or eye infection: excessive tearing, a burning sensation, cloudy or foggy vision that cannot be cleared by blinking, continuous redness of the eyes, feelings of scratchiness, general discomfort or pain. If any of these symptoms appears, remove the lenses. If the symptoms disappear after 24 hours, try the lenses again; if the symptoms persist or return, consult your eye doctor. Contact lenses are a great advance in corrective lenses, but they and the sensitive eyes behind them must be treated with extra caution if they are to become permanent working partners. ✳

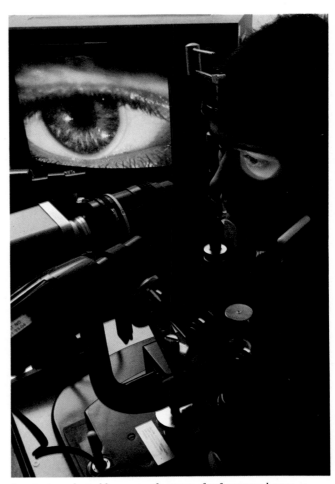

In a test conducted by a manufacturer of soft contact lenses, a television camera records the movement of a lens on a wearer's eye and projects an enlarged image of the eye on a screen. Researchers use this technique to improve the fit of lenses; if properly shaped, they will stay centered when the wearer blinks.

82

What's wrong with your eyes?

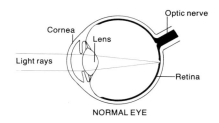

NORMAL EYE

The eyesight of most people is good enough so that—before age begins to take its inevitable toll—they can focus sharply on a nearby speck or distant star, see people across the room without distortion, and quickly spot objects off to one side. The eye can do all these things only if it has a smoothly curved cornea, a clear lens, a proper shape, strong muscles and a healthy retina firmly in place (drawing, above right). Any flaw in this system distorts, blurs or obscures the scene.

What the world looks like to people afflicted with common eye abnormalities is depicted in these specially made photographs; the drawings sketch each defect (indicated in red) and show how it can be corrected. The visual distortions described on these two pages are readily remedied with eyeglasses; the serious abnormalities explained on the following pages can also be treated, but may require surgery.

ASTIGMATISM

The photograph below exaggerates one kind of visual distortion caused by astigmatism. The stretching effect may be vertical, as in this case, or at any angle; the entire scene may also be blurred. This common optical error is usually accompanied by nearsightedness or farsightedness, and either of these defects worsens the warped vision.

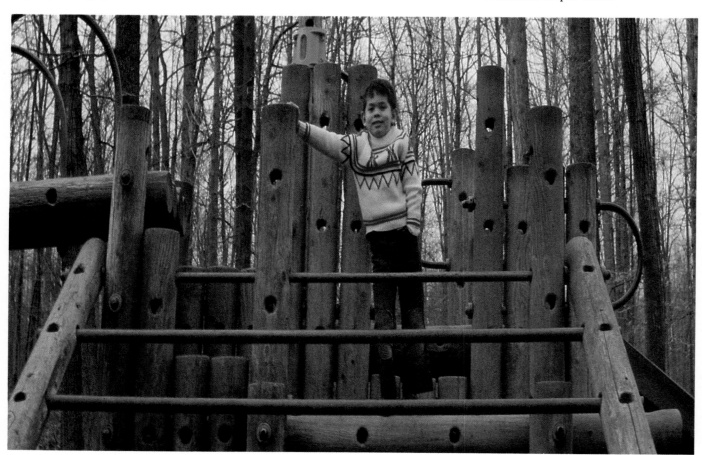

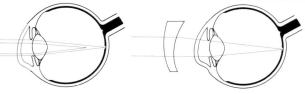

In astigmatism, a misshapen cornea (right) brings horizontal and vertical light rays into focus at different points—one (blue) on the retina and another (red) short of it. A cylindrical corrective lens (far right) focuses all the rays on the retina.

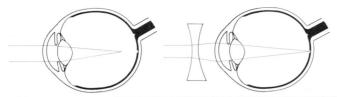

NEARSIGHTEDNESS

The view seen by a person with simple myopia, or nearsightedness, is similar to the one at right: The girl, a few feet away, appears clearly focused, the boy just behind her is fuzzy, and the background is almost a total blur. The cause may be an eyeball that is too long, a cornea that is too sharply curved or, in extreme cases, both.

Most nearsighted people notice the problem around the age of four, when the eyeball has grown enough to require a squint to compensate for the anomaly (partly closing the eye sharpens a fuzzy image just as a smaller opening in a camera lens improves sharpness). By the age of 25, the eyeball is shaped into its ultimate form and myopia progresses no further. Mainly a hereditary disorder passed from parents to children, nearsightedness is, for reasons unknown, most common among Asian people.

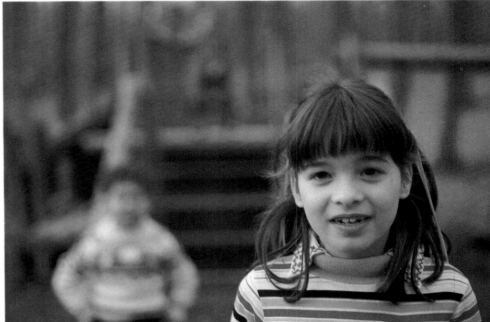

FARSIGHTEDNESS

The photograph at right depicts a scene as it would appear to a person with hyperopia, or farsightedness. The boy on the ladder is seen clearly, but the boy in the middle distance looks blurred and the girl in the foreground is barely recognizable. A short eyeball and an insufficiently curved cornea both contribute to the condition.

Farsightedness escapes detection in many young people because youthful eye muscles are strong enough to force the lens to compensate and bring near objects into focus; it is usually in middle age, when the muscles have lost some of their resilience, that the blurring becomes obvious.

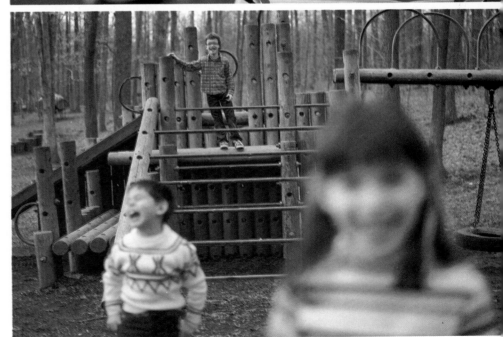

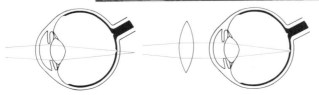

In a farsighted eye, the diverging light rays from nearby objects cannot be bent enough by the eye to converge them on the retina (far left). A convex lens (left) reduces divergence of the incoming rays so that the eye can finish the job.

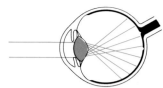

In the case of a cataract, light rays passing through the clouded lens (red) are scattered all over the retina instead of being brought to a focus. The result is a veiling of the field of vision, starting from the sides (below).

CATARACTS

To someone with cataracts, the world might resemble the blotchy scene of this photograph. Cataracts result when the lens of the eye, normally transparent as water, becomes unclear in spots or even totally opaque, obstructing part or all of the view.

Although cataracts affect some young people, they are an almost inevitable consequence of age. Anyone who lives to be 80 is virtually certain to develop them in one or both eyes, although fewer than 5 per cent of the cases need treatment. Even in elderly people, vision can be restored; removal of the lens provides a clear path for light, and eyeglasses then substitute for the natural lens in focusing an image.

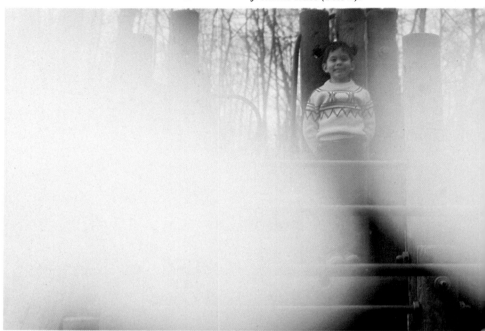

GLAUCOMA

If glaucoma is not treated promptly, side vision gradually disappears until the victim can see only what he looks at directly *(right)*. Glaucoma occurs when the system that provides and drains the fluid around the cornea goes off balance; fluid builds up, causing pressure inside the eye that kills fibers in the optic nerve, starting with those serving the edges of the retina and working inward.

Killed nerve fibers cannot be restored, but the damage can be prevented. Surgery can repair some defects in the fluid system, and pressure can be held in check with drugs that reduce the production of fluid or cause excess to drain away.

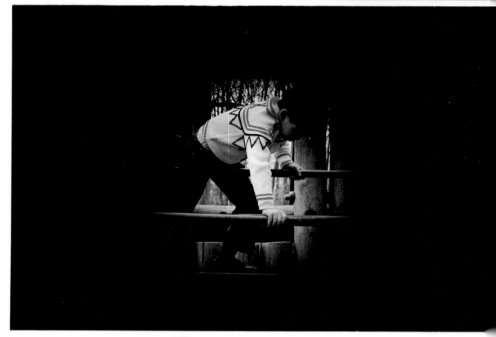

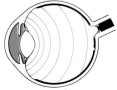

In glaucoma, pressure increases uniformly all through the inside of the eyeball but affects the optic nerve, at the back of the eye. It first destroys the nerve fibers that are involved in peripheral vision, but eventually can cut off all sight.

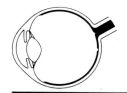 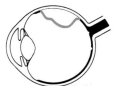

In the normal eye (far left), the retina is held securely against the inside of the eyeball. But if it pulls away from the wall of the eye (left), the part flapping downward is unable to record images, and the field of vision is reduced.

DETACHED RETINA

A healthy retina fits snugly against the back wall of the eyeball, pressed in place by the jelly-like fluid, called the vitreous humor, that fills the space between the lens and the back wall. If part of the retina comes loose, symptoms may show up as a blind spot in the view *(right)*, for the part of the retina that pulls away can no longer capture light rays and send an image to the brain.

If diagnosed in time, 90 per cent of detached retinas can be put back in place by any of several methods. In some cases the retina is literally spot-welded to the back wall of the eye by a laser beam.

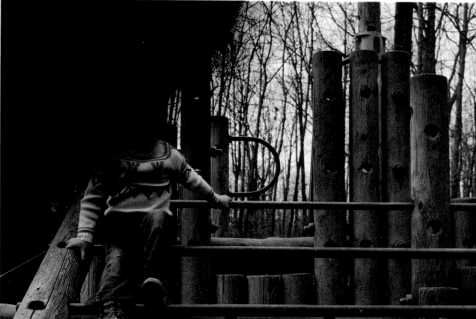

MACULAR DEGENERATION

The vision impairment caused by macular degeneration, the failure of a small region in the center of the retina, is exaggerated in this photograph; in most cases the blind spot is irregular and small. The macula, only about .06 inch across, contains the great majority of the cone cells, which provide sharp, color vision.

Any disease that afflicts the cones will leave just peripheral vision; the victim can see only out of the corners of the eye, and the view is fuzzy and lacking in color. Causes of macular degeneration include an inadequate blood supply to the retina, bleeding behind the macula, prolonged use of antimalaria drugs or injury to the retina. Until recently there was no cure. But now a simple treatment with a laser, approved for general use in 1982, is expected to prevent blindness in 90 per cent of the cases if begun within a few weeks after symptoms appear.

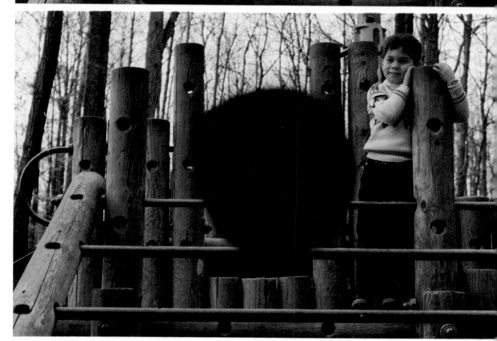

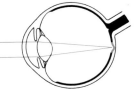

When the macula (red) is affected by disease or a wound, light rays still reach it normally, but it can no longer respond. The loss of its detailed vision—the sharp view gotten by looking straight at an object—is a severe handicap.

CHAPTER 4

Foiling the thieves of sight

Cataracts: lenses turned to agate
Victory over glaucoma
The marijuana treatment
Threats to the vulnerable retina
The key to cure—prompt action
Coping with blindness

Among the world's eye diseases, the greatest toll is exacted by trachoma, the work of a microscopic parasite called *trachoma chlamidia,* which invades the eyelid and inflames and scratches the cornea. It blinds two million people every year. Yet trachoma is practically unheard of in industrialized countries; modern sanitation has all but eliminated the parasite, and antibiotics have made the disease curable. Indeed, most of the other great eye ailments have been brought under control. Eye troubles arising from infections, once a major scourge, are, like trachoma, now prevented or cured. Today, the majority of serious eye maladies arise from the consequences of aging, and most of them can also be successfully treated.

Although serious eye diseases are more treatable than ever, they are more prevalent than ever. One reason for this paradox arises from a medical Catch-22: Because the major blinding diseases are, by and large, disorders of aging—68 per cent of the blind population is 65 or older—they have become more common as medicine has increased life expectancy. This fact alone would not make so much difference were it not for a distinctive characteristic of the worst thieves of sight: They are sneak thieves. They develop slowly and—to the victim—almost imperceptibly, causing no pain or noticeable disturbance of vision until the damage has been done. They can be detected early, however, by a doctor, and if caught at this stage rarely result in blindness. This is why regular eye examinations, particularly for the middle-aged and the elderly, are so essential.

Two of these insidious maladies are the major villains. Cataracts, which cloud the lenses and fog vision, are an almost inevitable consequence of aging; they afflict three fourths of all people past the age of 60, according to the National Society to Prevent Blindness. Glaucoma, an increase in internal eye pressure that attacks the optic nerve, affects at least two million Americans. These two diseases are readily remedied by surgery or drugs. Less controllable but fortunately much less common are a number of ailments, some arising from the aging process, that damage the light-sensitive lining of the eye, the retina.

Despite the allusion of its name to a waterfall, a cataract is not a watery curtain or film that falls across the surface of the lens—although many victims complain that their world looks as if seen through a waterfall. Rather, cataracts are the result of rearrangements in the structure of transparent protein molecules that make up the lens and the membrane that encloses it. The molecules lose their clarity because of changes in the way they transmit light. These molecules are normally small, but in cataracts they clump into aggregates 50 times their usual size, blocking and scattering light rays instead of focusing them on the receptor cells of the retina.

In a few cases the reasons for the molecular rearrangements are identifiable: heredity, diseases such as diabetes, or injuries. Some babies are born with cataracts because their mothers contracted German measles, syphilis or mumps during the first three months of pregnancy, upsetting the biochemical development of the fetal lens.

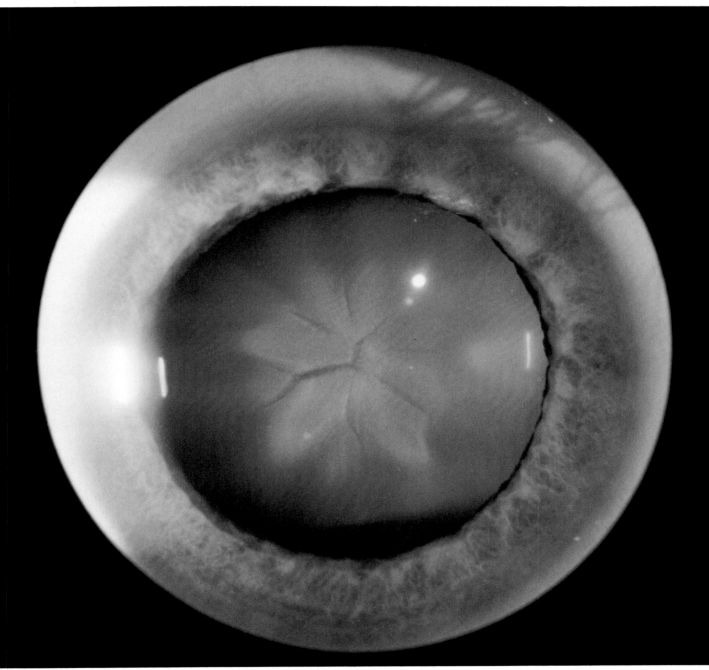

If a blow to the eye ruptures the capsule encasing the lens, the result may be a cataract like this one, a star-shaped cloud in the lens. The vision-obstructing pattern, which may form months after the injury, is different from the irregular cloudiness of the more common cataracts that develop with age. Both types are treated by surgical removal of the lens.

Radiation of many kinds can also damage the lens molecules, and this phenomenon has led to concern over danger from video screens—the TV-like displays on the consoles of computer terminals and word-processors, at which many people work day after day. The electronic devices that create the images on these screens are known to generate some X-rays, and some cases of cataracts have been blamed on exposure to them. However, government tests of a large number of video screens—including some that had been purposely damaged to disable their safety devices—indicated that, with few exceptions, none emitted more than a tenth the radiation permitted from television sets.

In nearly seven out of 10 cases of cataracts, the reasons for the lens-clouding molecular changes are unknown. Doctors view such cataracts as baffling mysteries of the aging process—the products of subtle, slow and irreversible changes in the composition of the lens. Indeed, such cataracts can develop for a period of 10 years or longer before they interfere significantly with vision. During that phase, as the cataract matures, vision may be almost normal. It may even improve: In a phenomenon known as second sight, some older people who have had poor near vision suddenly find themselves able to read fine print without glasses. This is the result of ongoing changes within the lens, which temporarily increase the ability of the lens to bend light and focus it on the retina. But second sight quickly vanishes as the maturing cataracts degrade all vision.

Cataracts: lenses turned to agate

Cataracts can develop in one eye or both. Because they often start at the center of the lens and grow outward, vision impairment frequently is noticed first in bright light, when the pupil is narrowest. Light passing through the center of the lens is scattered, often taking on a sunburst pattern. Nighttime driving frequently becomes difficult, because oncoming headlights turn the road into a blur. Glare, annoying under normal circumstances, takes on sight-paralyzing power. Eventually the ability to see under any conditions is compromised. Some light continues to penetrate the clouded lens, but colors and shapes become indistinguishable. ''Your

lenses turn into agate,'' said one 68-year-old Californian with cataracts in both eyes, ''and you are forced to look through stone.''

No one need live with lenses of agate. Although cataracts cannot be cured, the clouding of vision can be corrected. Repair always entails removal of the lens by surgery—a delicate but relatively simple procedure *(Chapter 5)*—and replacement with an artificial substitute. Occasionally the substitute is implanted directly into the eye at the time of the cataract surgery, but in three out of four cases, the replacement consists of contact lenses or spectacles that are prescribed after surgery.

The thick ''bottle-bottom'' lenses that are an unmistakable emblem of cataract repair were developed in the early 1900s by two European researchers—Dr. Moritz von Rohr, a physicist then working for the famous German lens maker Carl Zeiss, and Dr. A. Gullstrand, a Swedish ophthalmologist. Among the earliest to benefit from the thick lenses was the Impressionist painter Claude Monet, who, before his surgery in 1923, had been forced to restrict his painting to the hours around dawn and dusk, since the brightness of midday caused pain in his ailing eyes.

Although the spectacles work remarkably well—sight at the center of view usually is close to perfect—they cannot restore natural vision entirely, and they are very heavy. Because the new lens must be farther away from the retina than was the natural lens, the replacement must be very thick—as thick as one quarter of an inch at the center. Even when made of plastic, such lenses require unflattering heavy-duty frames that are tiring to wear.

More annoying than the weight are the optical effects introduced by thick lenses, which are so powerful they magnify objects 25 per cent or more. Such magnification alters depth perception, so that objects presumed to be at arm's length are found—after awkward groping—to be farther away. And because the lens is thicker at the center than it is at the sides, images suffer a progressive distortion: What is seen through the center of the lens is clear, although magnified, while what is seen through the edges is altered; straight lines, for example, may appear as curves. Perhaps most disturbing, however, are blind spots introduced in the intermediate range of vision—15 inches to 20 feet away, depending on the prescription. Again, lens thickness and curvature are at fault: The portion of the lens that in an ordinary pair of glasses would provide intermediate vision is tapered in cataract spectacles in such a way that light is bent excessively, entirely missing the retina. As a result, said one doctor, "Faces pop in and out of the blind area with the annoying insolence of a jack-in-the-box."

The experience of a fun-house view

Adjusting to this fun-house view of the world can take considerable time and patience. To provide more understanding counsel to patients, Miami ophthalmologist Dr. Robert C. Welsh decided to experience the visual effects himself not long ago. He devised a way to see as a cataract victim does. First Dr. Welsh placed on both his eyes a pair of special contact lenses; their purpose was to impose upon him the utter fuzziness that removal of both natural lenses imposes on a cataract patient. Then he fitted himself with a pair of cataract spectacles. "Vision was immediately remarkably clear," he said, "but everything was tremendously magnified, and all objects in the field of view seemed to swim back and forth with each turning of the eyes or with movement of the head. Vertical lines such as door jambs bowed out at the top and bottom when seen through the lens periphery. Through the spectacles everything seemed much closer than normal. People were much taller. In group conversation at two or three feet I was impressed by the fact that only two faces fitted into the stationary-head field of view."

Dr. Welsh found he had to alter movements to allow for the glasses' distortion. "The floor seemed much closer. My feet were missing: I had actually to bend my head forward about forty-five degrees to see them. It was necessary to walk with my legs apart, as on a rolling ship, to keep myself from falling." Even such accommodation did not prevent unpleasant sensations. "I walked down the hall to the elevator with relative ease except that the swimming back and forth of the field of view gave a nauseating feeling in the pit of my stomach. Outside on the pavement the basic instinct of

self-preservation made me turn my head rapidly back and forth to see who and what was where to avoid a collision. Crossing the street at the busy corner next to my medical building was horrifying—though I had crossed it for fifteen years—notwithstanding the special crossing light there for pedestrians only."

Dr. Welsh would have felt even more helpless had he simulated the vision of people who undergo a cataract operation in one eye only. They see double. One image is taken in through the normal eye, another—larger and more distorted—through the lensless eye. At first, the difference is more than the brain can assimilate. Confusion, loss of balance and headaches are frequent accompaniments in the postoperative period.

In time, however, most people adjust to cataract spectacles. If a cataract has been removed from only one eye, the adjustment frequently comes about by learning the awkward if perfectible technique of using the good eye for near vision, while suppressing or closing the lensless eye. The process is reversed for distant views, the lensless eye and the cataract glasses doing the work. If cataracts have been removed from both eyes, sight is best when the eyes are held straight and images are viewed through the center of the spectacle lenses. For reading and for seeing objects at the edges of the visual field, most patients experience less distortion and discomfort if they turn their heads and not merely their eyes.

The short-term adjustments—and long-term visual distortions—imposed by cataract spectacles can be largely avoided by using contact lenses. Because a contact lens is located just a layer of tears away from the eyeball itself, it is hardly any farther from the retina than the original lens it replaces. It introduces little magnification—only about 8 per cent. Consequently depth and distance perception are less affected. Because the contact lens moves with the eye, it produces much less distortion at the edges of the view than do cataract glasses, and the field of vision is much greater. Even a person with one normal eye and one equipped with a cataract contact lens can gaze on the world through two nearly matched eyes.

Cataract contact lenses, for all their advantages, suffer the same drawbacks as ordinary contacts; many people find them uncomfortable or difficult to manipulate. The lens must also be several times thicker and heavier than ordinary contacts, and consequently is more likely to slip downward from its proper position on the cornea. And in rare instances, the cataract surgery may leave the corneal surface with a bulge that a contact lens cannot fit.

Victory over glaucoma

The success of modern treatment of cataracts is equaled by the victories doctors have won over glaucoma. This disease, characterized by abnormally high pressure inside the eyeball, attacks one in every 50 Americans over the age of 35. Because it is essentially symptomless until its late stages, half of those stricken do not know they have it. Unaware of their potentially disabling illness, they do not get the treatment that can halt progress of the ailment. "Most other diseases are revealed by pain or other disturbance," wrote Dr. Ben Esterman, a Manhattan eye surgeon, but "a person suffering from glaucoma may not be aware of trouble until he has lost much of the sight in one eye and some of the sight in the other." Glaucoma, although almost always treatable, remains the leading cause of blindness in the United States.

Glaucoma is an accumulation of aqueous humor, the clear fluid that fills the chambers between the cornea and the lens *(page 33)*. The aqueous humor is secreted continuously by an organ called the ciliary body, located alongside the lens. Normally, excess aqueous humor drains out of the eye through tiny ducts, called the trabecular meshwork, that are nestled deep in the V-shaped recesses where the cornea curves to meet the iris. From the trabecular meshwork the fluid then passes through a network of drainage canals into the bloodstream for disposal. In glaucoma, aqueous humor builds up because too much is produced or, far more often, because the excess fails to drain properly.

The drainage failure can occur in two ways. In rare instances, the problem arises abruptly: The V-shaped recess is either abnormally narrow at birth, or it is pinched shut by infection or by a sudden, involuntary dilation of the pupil; eye muscles then may seal off the trabecular meshwork so that pressure builds quickly.

But in nine out of 10 cases of glaucoma, the drainage clog comes on slowly, and so does the pressure. For reasons that seem associated with heredity (people with relatives who have had glaucoma are four times as likely as others to get the disease) the drainage ducts and canals deteriorate with age. As fluid accumulates and pressure builds—whether slowly or quickly—the fibers of the optic nerve and the capillaries that nourish them are squeezed. Crushed and starved for blood, the nerve fibers die.

In gradually developing glaucoma, the outermost fibers die first, those at the core later. Because the fibers serving peripheral vision lie on the outer layers of the optic nerve and those serving central vision lie within the core, the first effect on sight noticed is loss of peripheral vision. The ability to see things off to one side—essential to driving safely—will begin to fail. Without treatment, the view will gradually narrow down to "tunnel vision," so that only the center of a scene can be observed. Total blindness can follow swiftly.

A tragic example of glaucoma's effects on peripheral vision was recounted in a 1977 book by Manhattan ophthalmologist Ben Esterman. A 55-year-old chauffeur with an excellent record for safe driving was suddenly involved in two auto accidents in rapid succession. After the first, a cursory examination by motor vehicle officials found no eye trouble. The man's central vision was perfect. Unfortunately, the eye test did not evaluate side vision. Only after the second accident, in which a child on a bicycle was killed, did the chauffeur consult Dr. Esterman, who quickly discovered glaucoma, far advanced in the right eye and beginning in the left. Side vision in the right eye was almost gone. "The child he had killed," reported Dr. Esterman, "was riding a bicycle to the right side of his car. He never saw the child until he had hit him."

Such tragedies are unnecessary, for diagnosis and treatment of chronic glaucoma is generally simple and reliable. A regular visit to an eye doctor is the first line of defense. Most experts advise an examination once every two years after the 40th birthday—or once a year and starting earlier, if a close blood relative has had the ailment.

The ophthalmologist checks for glaucoma by measuring

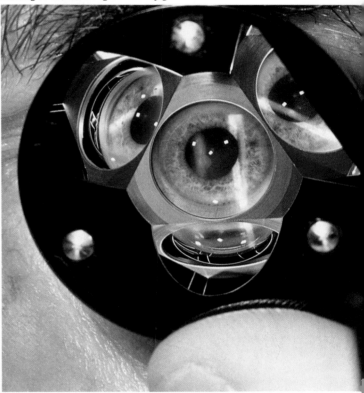

A combination of lenses, prisms and mirrors in an instrument called a gonioscope looks into this eye from several directions at once. It reveals the retina (reddish circle, center) but is mainly used to check the angle where iris and cornea meet (upper left). A narrow angle there may impede drainage of eye fluids, leading to the blinding ailment of glaucoma.

eye pressure. He does so with a tonometer—any of several types based on one invented in 1905 by Dr. Hjalmar August Schiötz, an Oslo eye doctor. The device squeezes the eyeball, employing a principle not unlike that used when you press into a bicycle tire with your thumb to judge how much it is inflated. The doctor first prepares the eye with a couple of drops of topical anesthetic and instructs the patient to fix his eyes on some distant object. The doctor next places the tonometer against the cornea's surface and releases a plunger or a puff of air to indent the cornea. How much the cornea is depressed by this push, indicated by a scale on the plunger, reveals pressure inside the eye: The less the indentation, the higher the pressure.

If glaucoma is suggested by excessive eye pressure, specialized tests follow to confirm the diagnosis and to determine the extent of the damage. Central and peripheral vision are assessed with reading charts and exercises. The drainage structures of the eye are examined with a gonioscope, a mirror-and-lens instrument that gauges the angle of the V-shaped recesses leading to the ducts. The doctor then looks inside the eye to check for damage to the optic nerve, visible at the point where it terminates in a disklike structure on the retina. An abnormally pale, depressed disk—"cupping"— is a certain sign of nerve damage.

Before the mid-19th Century, glaucoma was incurable. In the 1850s, however, a German surgeon, Dr. Albrecht von Graefe, devised a procedure called iridectomy, in which he cut a tiny hole in the iris, creating an artificial passageway to help fluid drain out of the eye *(Chapter 5)*. Two decades later another German physician, Dr. Ludwig Laqueur, found a simpler treatment. He discovered that the compound physostigmine, obtained from a West African bean, could constrict the pupil, thereby opening the eye drains and lowering eyeball pressure. Since then most cases of glaucoma have been controlled with medicine rather than surgery. Control, however, has not meant cure: Glaucoma medicines, usually in the form of eye drops, must be administered day in, day out, by the patient for the rest of his life.

Drugs that are now used to treat chronic glaucoma fall into two basic categories: those called miotics, including physo-

stigmine and the more recently developed pilocarpine, which improve the drainage of fluids out of the eye; and those that inhibit fluid production in the first place, namely the adrenergics and the carbon anhydrase inhibitors. The difference in approach can be compared to raising the bridge or lowering the river; in opposite ways, the two sorts of drugs deliver essentially the same result.

Miotic eye drops are the standard choice because they have fewer side effects than the other glaucoma drugs. The most frequently prescribed miotic is pilocarpine, a derivative of the South American jaborandi tree, which was first used in the late 19th Century. Some people experience blurred vision or a burning sensation in the eyes soon after putting the drops in—side effects of the severe constriction of their pupils that lets trapped aqueous fluid flow out. The many glaucoma

In a test of marijuana as a glaucoma remedy, Keith Green of the Medical College of Georgia uses a special tonometer (page 72) to measure fluid pressure in the eye of a rabbit that has been treated with drops containing a cannabis compound. Certain chemicals in the drug control the abnormally high pressure of glaucoma, but they may have other, undesirable effects.

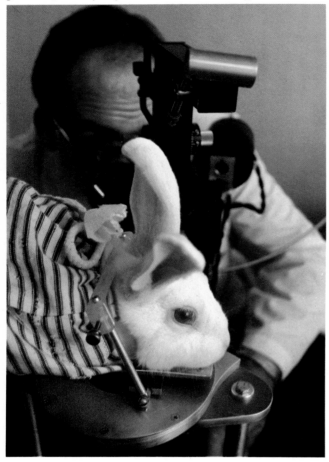

victims who also suffer from developing cataracts may experience a slight dimming of vision in poor light, again the consequence of narrowed pupils.

Pilocarpine is also available in a time-release capsule. A very small, drug-impregnated soft plastic disk, it is slipped under the lower eyelid. It remains there, continuously releasing measured amounts of medicine into the eye, for seven days, and is then replaced with a fresh insert. Because the amounts of pilocarpine at work at any one time are extremely small, the side effects of the more potent drops are avoided.

If a miotic drug cannot control eyeball pressure, adrener-

gics, also in eye-drop form, frequently are prescribed. Epinephrine derivatives are the most widely used. Adrenergic drops work, in effect, as a depressant on the ciliary body, relaxing it and slowing its production of aqueous humor. Carbon anhydrase inhibitors—acetazolamide is the most widely used—produce a similar slowing of aqueous humor production, but by mechanisms that are not well understood.

The marijuana treatment

Still another, very controversial remedy for glaucoma is marijuana. In the late 1960s, as marijuana use was on the upswing, doctors noticed that smokers typically exhibited red eyes. This phenomenon suggested that other, unseen ophthalmological effects might be taking place. In 1972, Dr. Robert S. Hepler and two colleagues at the University of California at Los Angeles documented one of them: They found that marijuana lowered eyeball pressure in 12 research volunteers by an average of 25 per cent. None of Dr. Hepler's subjects suffered from glaucoma, but subsequent research with glaucoma patients, by Dr. Hepler and others, turned up similar pressure-reducing results.

Dozens of studies followed this work. ''All of them,'' said Professor Keith Green, a marijuana researcher at the Medical College of Georgia in Augusta, ''have confirmed, over and over again, that when a marijuana cigarette is smoked, or when certain of the plant's main active ingredients—principally cannabinoids, and delta-9-tetrahydrocannabinol in particular—are ingested in capsule form or by injection, that pressure in the eyeballs will fall.''

Such evidence has persuaded some legal authorities to make marijuana available—through physicians operating with special permits—to selected glaucoma patients. One such patient, Robert C. Randall of Washington, D.C., made headlines in 1976 when he challenged his arrest for growing marijuana in a pot on his balcony. Randall claimed that marijuana was the only drug that controlled his glaucoma. The Superior Court of the District of Columbia sided with Randall, granting him the right to smoke the weed under a doctor's supervision—but not to grow it.

Unfortunately, while marijuana lowers pressure in the

eye, it also raises heart rate, interferes with mental and motor functions and, if smoked heavily over time, is thought to damage the lungs. Thus, Professor Green suggested that ''marijuana, as a smoked weed, has no potential as a glaucoma drug. However, if we can isolate or synthesize pure cannabinoids that lower pressure in the eye but do not produce adverse side effects, we may have a potentially useful glaucoma drug.''

Threats to the vulnerable retina

Although cataracts and glaucoma are the serious eye diseases most frequently diagnosed in the United States, accounting for about a third of all blindness, another group of eye ailments, less common but much more difficult to treat, are greater thieves of sight. These are disorders of the light-sensitive retina lining the back of the eye; they cause almost half the total cases of blindness, although they afflict only 1/100 as many people as glaucoma and cataracts. In all these ailments, light-sensitive cells of the retina die, sometimes because their nourishment is cut off, sometimes because the retina pulls away from the inner wall of the eyeball, sometimes for no identifiable reason.

The retina is so vulnerable because of its extreme complexity. It has been termed ''the ultimate level of sophistication in the evolution of biologic tissue'' by Dr. David Miller, chief of ophthalmology at Beth Israel Hospital in Boston, who said, ''It can both detect a few quanta of light and process a complex visual scene,'' transmitting up to half a billion pieces of information every second.

''Nature's price for such complexity,'' continued Dr. Miller, ''is rapid energy turnover.'' The retina consumes oxygen and the body's principal fuel, the blood sugar glucose, at higher rates than any other tissue. Because these substances are supplied by the circulatory system, said Dr. Miller, ''the amount of blood-flow per unit time, per gram of tissue, is also the greatest in the body.'' Any disorder that interferes with this blood supply can do severe damage.

Diabetes—the inability of the body to produce energy by processing sugars and starches—is just such a disease. Its principal visual complication, diabetic retinopathy, is today the most frequently diagnosed disorder of the retina: About 5,000 new cases are found each year. It has become common because treatment for diabetes is now so successful. Before the advent of insulin therapy in the 1920s, diabetic retinopathy was virtually unknown—diabetics died before the disease could damage their eyes. Nowadays, according to a study by Dr. Arnall Patz, of Johns Hopkins University, about 70 per cent of diabetics who have the disease for 15 years will suffer diabetic retinopathy; among those who have diabetes for 25 years or more, the incidence is 90 to 95 per cent.

Diabetes damages blood vessels. Capillaries, the smallest and especially numerous in the retina, are hardest hit. In diabetic retinopathy, they change shape and their walls weaken; soon they begin to leak the clear, nutrient-laden serum of blood. Some vessels collapse or pinch shut altogether. In time the retina swells with fluid, tissues die of oxygen deprivation and vision blurs.

As retinopathy advances, new blood vessels develop to replace the damaged old ones. But the new vessels do not grow normally: They reach into the interior of the eye, into the vitreous humor itself. Even more fragile than the capillaries they replace, these newcomers bleed easily. The least damage to the eye can cause massive bleeding that suffuses the vitreous with blood, blocking the passage of all but the very brightest light. In time this blood may be reabsorbed into the bloodstream, just as the black and blue of a skin bruise will gradually fade, but in the retina, scar tissue often forms. When the scar tissue begins to contract, as it typically does in healing, it can wrench the retina from its normal position on the inner wall of the eye. Severe visual impairment and blindness are possible outcomes. Indeed, more than 30,000 Americans are blind because of diabetic retinopathy.

Detachment of the retina, the most dangerous result of diabetic retinopathy, can also strike people who have never suffered from diabetes. Normally the retina is firmly anchored inside the eye in two places: on the periphery, where it connects to an underlying layer that supplies it with nourishment, and at the center, where it grows into the optic nerve. Everywhere else it is held against the inner wall of the eye largely by the pressure of the vitreous humor, in much the same way that an inner tube is held snug against the inner wall of a tire by air pressure. If a tiny hole appears in an inner tube, the tube will separate from the tire wall. The same thing can happen to a retina. Part of it may simply pull loose, or it may tear, or it may do both. Either kind of damage can precede or initiate the other. One eye or both can be affected.

Retinal detachment can be caused not only by diabetes but also by aging or, sometimes, by a blow, an infection, a hemorrhage, a tumor, or an inherited disposition toward poor retinal adhesion. In a susceptible individual, violent coughing, sneezing or extreme physical exertion can knock loose part of the retina. Even severe nearsightedness, the result of an exaggeratedly long eyeball, can increase vulnerability, overstretching the retina so that it pulls loose easily. When the retina becomes unstuck, some blood gets into the vitreous humor and vision begins to suffer. The extent of the loss depends upon where the disruption occurs. If it is toward the outer edge of the retina, which provides peripheral vision, little change may be noticed. If, on the other hand, it occurs near the center of the retina—the part responsible for sharp central sight—detachment brings major disruption of vision.

The most frequent symptom is a blurring of peripheral vision, as though a curtain or permanent shadow has obscured a corner of the eye. Less reliable indicators are spots and light flashes, which occur frequently in eyes that are perfectly normal; many spots are "floaters"—strands of tissues or clumps of blood cells that have found their way into the vitreous humor but are soon reabsorbed. However, if the problem persists for more than a day or so, an eye examination is called for.

Central rather than peripheral vision is affected by another disease of the retina, macular degeneration. It develops when the wear and tear of aging damages the blood vessels serving the sharp-seeing central segment of the retina, the macula, causing it to separate from an underlying layer of tissue called the pigment epithelium. "The single-cell layer of pigment epithelium," reported Dr. David Miller of Beth Israel Hospital in Boston in 1979, "appears to be the key to the health of the retinal elements in the macula, regulating the transfer of nutrients and removing waste products." Unless treated within a few weeks, this disease generally causes loss of central vision, first in one eye and then in the other, although peripheral vision usually is retained in both eyes.

Blindness caused by macular degeneration, by detached retinas, or by the leaky blood vessels of diabetes is readily prevented today; one technique is spot welding with a laser beam *(Chapter 5)*. "In the 1930s," noted the New York City ophthalmologist, Dr. Ben Esterman, "an eye with retinal detachment was almost certain to remain blind. Fewer than one per cent could be cured. Now, after years of research, surgeons, using modern discoveries in physics and engineering, can cure over 95 per cent of detachments."

The key to cure—prompt action
Cure depends, however, on catching the ailment at an early stage. And the first signs of impending damage to the retina are not always easy to detect. Subtle changes that foretell deterioration may be missed by physicians who are not intimately familiar with the symptoms. The difficulty of recognizing retinal disease was demonstrated in a study made in 1981 by Dr. William G. Tsiaras of the University of Pennsylvania. He asked a group of 23 physicians to examine the eyes of patients who suffered from diabetic retinopathy but whose ailment was unknown to the examining doctors. The internists in the group of physicians missed more than half of the cases; diabetes specialists failed to detect one third, and even the general ophthalmologists overlooked one tenth. Only three ophthalmologists specializing in retinal diseases identified every case of retinopathy.

The technique used to examine diabetic retinopathy and many other retinal disorders is fluorescein angiography, which produces sharp pictures of seepage from retinal blood vessels. The clear fluid that oozes out of damaged vessels in the eye often is invisible to even the most sophisticated examining device; but when a dye called fluorescein is injected into a vein, the network of retinal capillaries can be seen. Fluorescein glows a brilliant green color when struck by blue light. The dye flows promptly—within 10 seconds or so—into the blood vessels of the eye and leaks out through

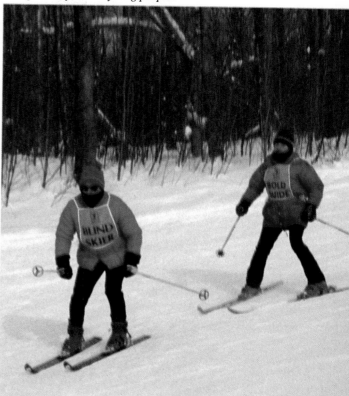

Unable to see but gliding freely down a Vermont slope, George Lovely (left) is guided by a volunteer ski instructor with an organization called Blind Outdoor Leisure Development (BOLD), which sponsors recreational activities for the blind. Lovely lost his vision to retinitis pigmentosa, a rare, blinding disease that generally strikes young people.

any holes that may be present, its glow in blue light revealing the location of the leaks. Even microscopic seepage shows up, permitting the prompt treatment that promises cure.

Regrettably, similar progress cannot be reported in the treatment of the potentially blinding retinal disorder called retinitis pigmentosa. Its causes are mysterious and little can be done to repair the damage it does.

Like macular degeneration, retinitis pigmentosa also involves the pigment epithelium. But that is the only similarity. The pigment provides vision by responding to light with a chemical change; it must then be regenerated, or returned to its light-sensitive chemical form, to maintain vision. This regeneration process deteriorates in retinitis pigmentosa, and the failure is first noticed in night vision, since seeing in dim light requires the most pigment. The retinal cells that contain the most pigment and thus are most important in night vision are the rods, which are most concentrated near the edge of the retina and serve as well for peripheral vision. Thus, ability to see to the side is also impaired. Eventually the whole retina shuts down.

No treatment has won general acceptance, although Soviet physicians claimed that injections of an extract of yeast, called Encad, at least halted the deterioration in some cases. Its value was not confirmed, however, in follow-up studies reported in 1982 by American physicians. Dr. Eliot Berson, an expert in retinitis pigmentosa at the Massachusetts Eye and Ear Infirmary in Boston, examined seven patients who had traveled to Moscow for Encad treatments. He found ''no beneficial effect,'' and reported that three of the seven suffered further deterioration of vision.

Retinitis pigmentosa is inherited and generally strikes its victims before they are 10 years old. But the onset can occur considerably later. Gordon Gund, a financier, experienced the first symptoms of retinitis pigmentosa when he was 25: ''I had difficulty walking on Wall Street, leaving the bank at night. I'd run into people because I wouldn't see them. I had trouble in darkened rooms. When I took customers from the bank to restaurants, we'd walk to the table and, before I'd even touched a drink, I'd bump into waitresses and tables. I found myself constantly apologizing.'' He continued, ''In the final stages I didn't know from one day to the next how much vision I'd have.'' By the time he was 30 Gordon Gund lost his vision altogether. One of the last things he saw was the face of his newborn son.

Coping with blindness

For people with retinitis pigmentosa, or for those blinded by accidents or born with such serious defects as damaged optic nerves, there is little that ophthalmology can do. Lost sight can seldom be restored; nonexistent vision can rarely be remedied.

But blindness is mercifully rare and rarely complete. Barely half a million Americans are legally blind; that is, their sight cannot be corrected to better than 20/200—the top line on a standard eye chart—or their field of vision is less than 20 degrees at its widest. But of that number, about 75 per cent have 20/200 vision. Many of these people—and others with less severely impaired vision—manage daily life by using special eyeglasses, lighting devices and other aids *(below)*.

For the remaining percentage of legally blind people, who at best can see only shades of light and dark, methods and devices for coping abound. Some are traditional and familiar; others are products of the computer age.

Even such an ancient device as a cane—still the most useful aid for the blind—can be improved. During World War II, Dr. Richard E. Hoover, working at the U.S. Army center for blinded veterans at Valley Forge, Pennsylvania, devised changes that added to the cane's utility. He lengthened it, giving it a scanning arc of five feet to the front and

sides, and he made it lighter and slimmer. Today, a typical blind person's cane, made of fiberglass, is hollow, weighs between one and two ounces and, at its handle, is about the diameter of a quarter—light and narrow enough for even the most delicate of hands. With such canes or with guide dogs, even the totally blind can generally get around on their own. New devices that use sound waves or laser beams to help blind people find their way *(Chapter 6)* promise to supplement these traditional aids.

New developments are more important in helping the blind work at their jobs, greatly expanding the applications of braille, the alphabet of raised dots that can be read by touch. The American Foundation for the Blind devised a braille electronic calculator to serve in bookkeeping. A more recent development has been the so-called talking calculator *(page*

Special helps for faltering eyes

The old notion that people with failing vision can "save" their eyes by not using them has been turned completely around: Now, doctors recommend a variety of aids to help patients make the most of their remaining vision. Surprisingly, about three out of four people considered legally blind—vision measured as poorer than 20/200—have enough eyesight remaining to benefit from the types shown here.

These aids fall into two basic categories: optical aids, such as magnifiers or oversized print, which enlarge the view; and tactile aids, which use raised bumps or lines to help people feel their way through tasks. Most are intended to ease the close work that troubles the visually handicapped. They can restore the ability to hold a job, go to school or take part in a sociable game of cards.

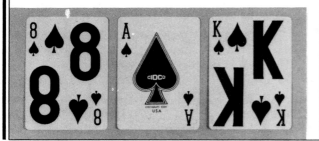

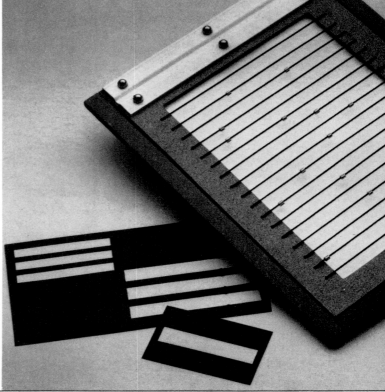

"Jumbo" cards are standard size but display enlarged symbols, and substitute letters for pictures of king, queen and jack. Each suit is in a different color—clubs are blue, not black like spades, and diamonds are green, not red like hearts.

Writing aids use raised forms to keep penmanship in line. A letter-sized guide has a lift-up frame crisscrossed by elastic cords marking off straight lines on paper placed beneath; small beads slide along the cords to indicate the writer's place. Stencils that fit over an envelope (left) or a receipt (bottom) have cut-outs where addresses and signatures belong.

143), which turns numbers into spoken words. Several different electronic devices enable blind people to read ordinary print. A miniature camera scans the printed page; the impulses are then picked up by a computer that recognizes the letters by their shape. The computer then processes the information and either transmits it to the reader by means of touch signals or generates the sounds of the words.

With the help of such inventions, blindness need not be an insurmountable handicap. Charles Kalb, who transcribes medical records at Johns Hopkins Hospital in Baltimore, recently said, ''I know normal people who are much more handicapped than I. They feel sorry for themselves. That is the greatest handicap.'' For financier Gordon Gund, the busy life he led before he lost his sight was not lost with vision. He continued to run his own investment firm, serve on the board

of directors of a half-dozen corporations and act as chief executive officer of the Minnesota North Stars hockey team; he became a trustee of the preparatory school from which he had been graduated, and helped found the National Retinitis Pigmentosa Foundation. He did not forgo athletics, continuing to swim, ski and play his favorite sport, hockey. ''They like to put me in the goal,'' he said with a laugh. ''I'm what every hockey player has always dreamed of shooting at—a blind goaltender.''

Eventually a goaltender blinded by retinitis pigmentosa should become an even rarer phenomenon. Research projects supported by organizations such as the one founded by Gordon Gund are uncovering the causes of retinitis pigmentosa, and even that disease may be added to the long list of those that have been conquered. ✺

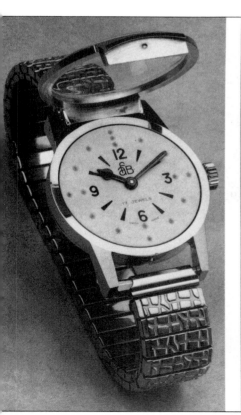

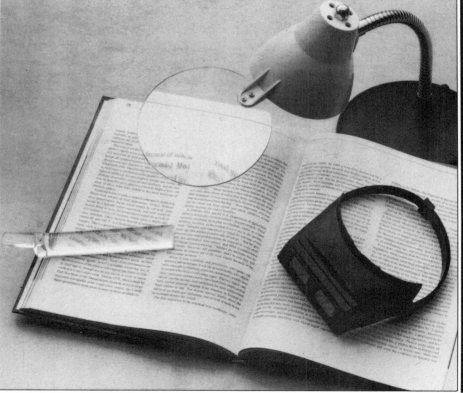

A wrist watch with a hinged crystal allows those with low vision to feel the time. Fingertips locate the long, plain minute hand and the shorter, arrow-tipped hour hand and identify hours by raised dots: Three dots mark 12 o'clock.

Among the many magnifiers that enlarge details for easier recognition are the three pictured above. The clear plastic bar at left lies flat on a page and covers two lines at a time; the high-intensity lamp fitted with a swiveling glass and the binocular magnifier that fastens around the head like goggles are especially useful because they free both hands for tasks.

A man who sees by memory and feel

Chatting with a fellow commuter as he rides the bus home from work, the man at right in most ways leads a perfectly typical life—as husband, father and breadwinner. Only the white cane gives Gordon Edwards away. He became blind at the age of 15 months after a bout of meningitis, a grave inflammation of membranes enclosing the brain.

Gordon Edwards is matter-of-fact about his handicap. Having no conception of what vision is like, he spends no more time yearning for it than a deep-sea dweller might spend coveting wings. "Sight is relative," he explained. "If you don't have it, you don't miss it." His family neither pitied nor pampered him during his childhood on their small farm in Kentucky, and he developed an exceptional memory and sense of touch to serve as substitute eyes.

These strengths give him an edge in his work for Cincinnati's giant soap manufacturer, Procter and Gamble. Assigned to the data center's "help desk," he answers phone calls from people who encounter problems while using computer facilities at more than 200 branch centers. A number of electronic devices aid him *(overleaf)*, transforming the light signals or print-outs he cannot see into forms he can feel or hear. But his most valuable tools are his listening and recall skills. "When a question arises," said Edwards' supervisor, "he quite often knows the answer as well as a book might."

When Gordon Edwards leaves work for the day, he rides a bus that stops just in front of his house—he and his wife Kathy went househunting with that need in mind. Kathy Edwards, because of a birth injury, has another kind of handicap—difficulty coordinating certain muscles. As a result, the couple works in tandem to accomplish many household tasks, using her eyes to guide his hands. When they brought their first baby home from the hospital, it was father who changed the first diaper with mother's guidance.

Proud of his competence and independence, Gordon Edwards bristles when people treat him as though he were an invalid—or invisible—because he is blind. "If I stop by a bar for a drink, I do not much appreciate someone getting up and giving me his seat and moving away," he said. "I do appreciate it if someone says 'Hey, there's an empty seat four places down.' And then let me find it on my own."

Their white canes signaling their handicap, Gordon Edwards and a blind neighbor share a bus seat for the commute home. The two are engaged in a favorite pastime— friendly betting on football games.

PHOTOGRAPHS BY GORDON BAER

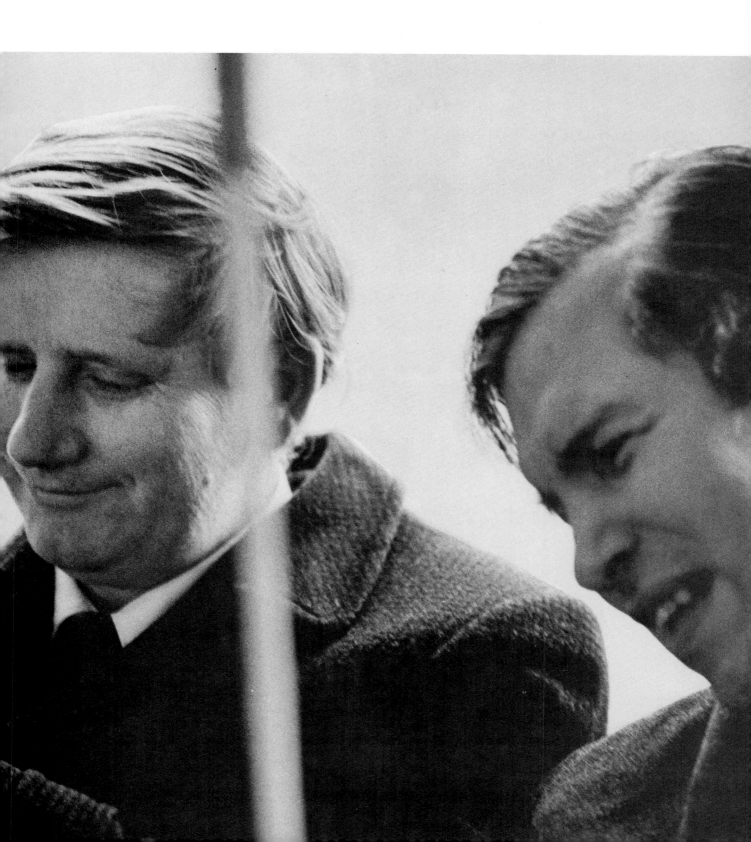

An office wired for work without sight

The computer terminal by Gordon Edwards' desk has been adapted with a brailling attachment (foreground). When he keys in messages, the computer's response is translated into braille on paper tape.

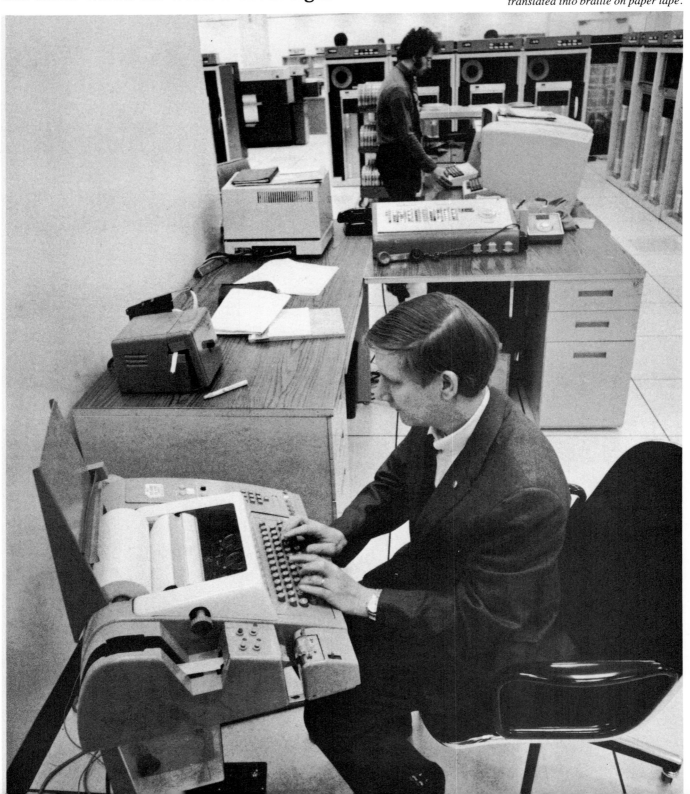

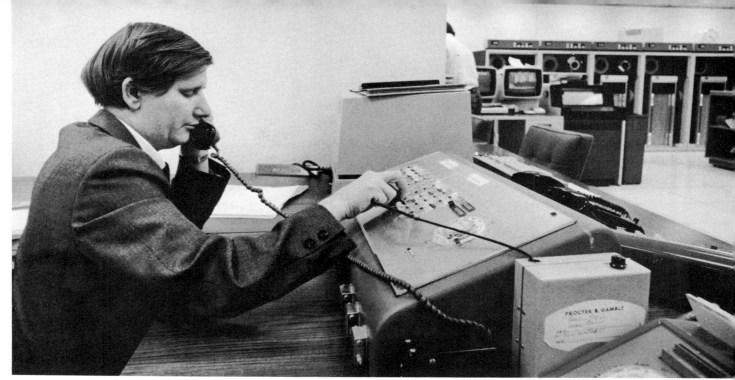

To answer telephone calls from computer users, Gordon
Edwards finds the calling line on the switchboard by detecting its
flashing signal with the light-sensitive wand in his hand. The
wand, connected to a control (foreground), emits a shrill tone
when it is centered over the lighted button of an incoming call,
telling Edwards which line to answer.

Gordon Edwards uses an Optacon to read printed material.
With his right hand he scans the page with a probe containing a
tiny television camera that converts the image of each letter
into an electronic message. His left hand monitors a grid in the
main unit, where the electronic signals activate tiny rods that
press the shape of the letter onto a fingertip.

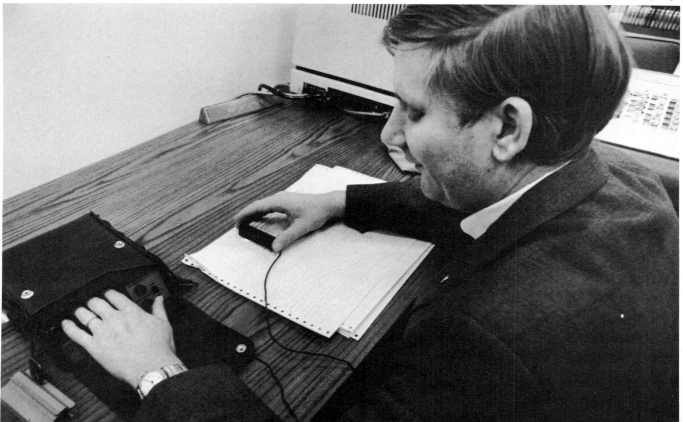

The challenge of getting from here to there

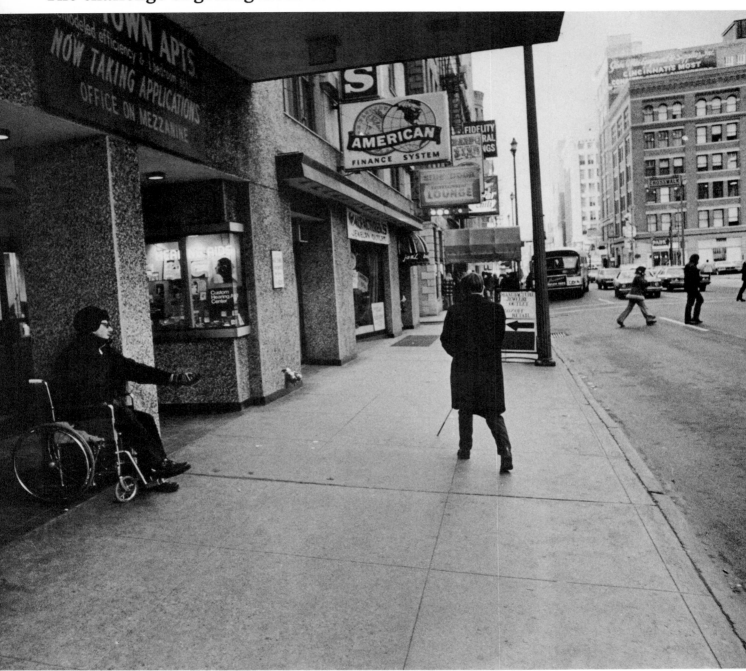

*As he walks the familiar three blocks from office to bus stop,
Gordon Edwards heeds a caution from a wheelchair-bound man,
a neighborhood figure who directs Edwards back to the center
of the sidewalk—his steps had begun veering toward the curb.*

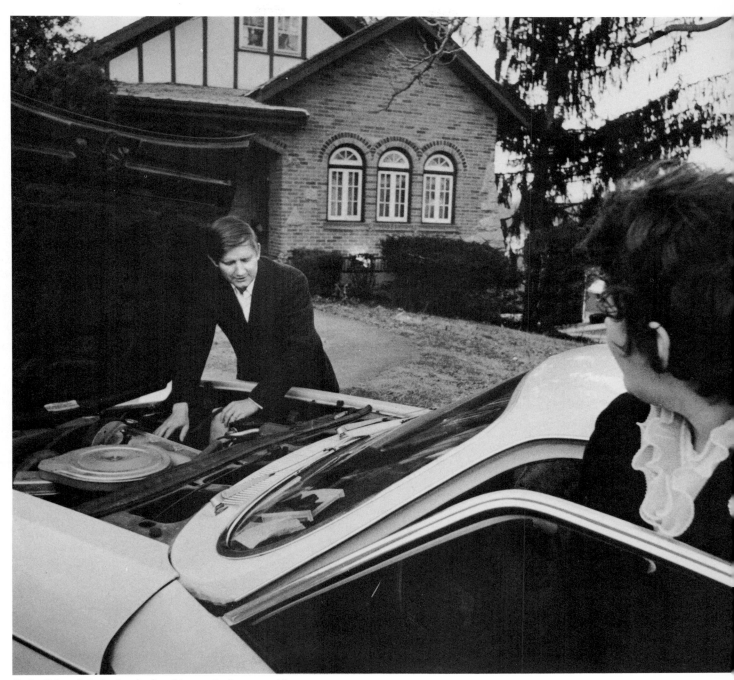

Kathy Edwards helps her husband locate the battery cables on their stalled car—jiggling them sometimes improves contact so that the engine will start. Aside from simple maintenance, Gordon's automotive role is limited to riding as a passenger. This, he pointed out, is the greatest frustration of being blind—his inability to drive a car.

Sharing the work—and play—at home

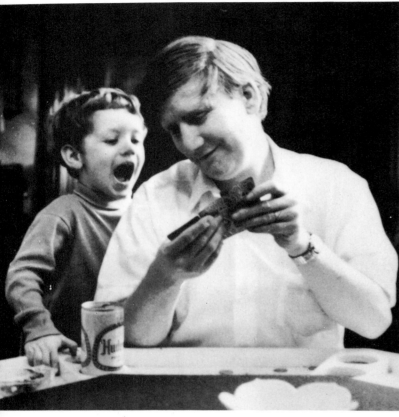

Three-year-old Brian and his father bridge a sensory gap to share a moment of glee over a good poker hand: The son sees the cards, the father feels them. A longtime lover of the game, Gordon Edwards plays with sighted friends by modifying a regular deck. He impresses the appropriate symbols on each card with his brailler, a punching device with six keys and a space bar.

Replacing a light bulb in the children's playroom, Edwards balances on a stool under the fixture, which he can locate by memory. ''No big deal,'' he insisted. He routinely does the dishes and peels vegetables, and once, in a burst of ambition, he and a partially sighted friend renovated an entire wall of kitchen cabinets.

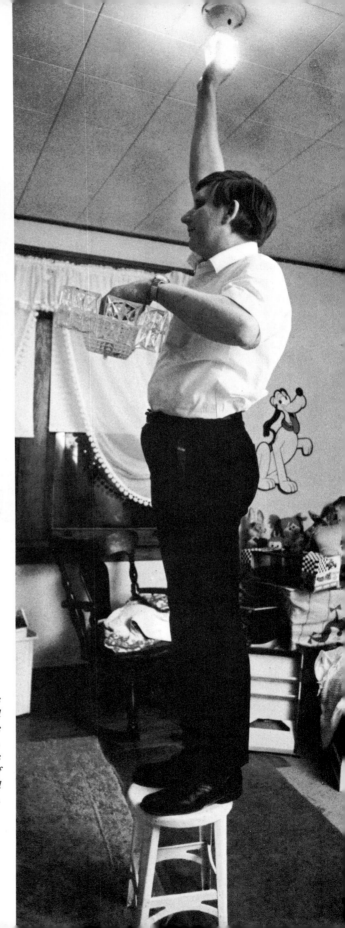

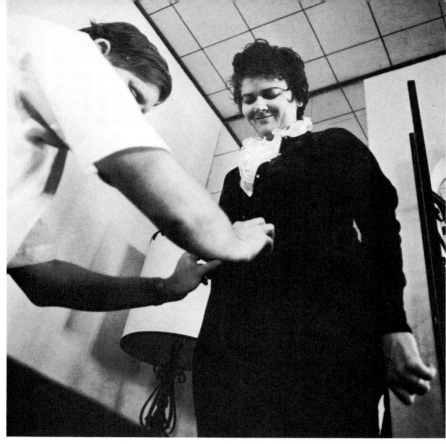

In a hurried moment, Kathy asks Gordon to help button her dress—a cumbersome task for her stiff fingers. A social worker by profession, she helps train medical students and interns to guide disabled patients in adjusting to their handicaps.

Kathy selects a shirt for Gordon so that he will wear clothes of coordinated colors. Part of her evening routine is hanging his next day's outfit on the closet door—shirt, then slacks and suit jacket with tie tucked in the pocket. She also buys his clothes.

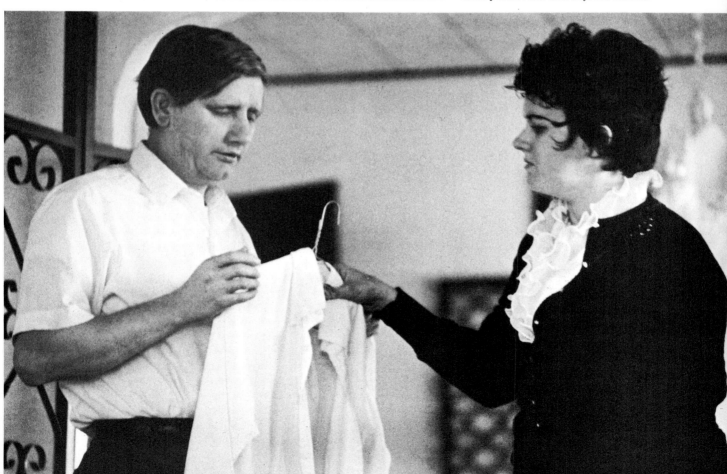

Fatherly love conveyed by touch

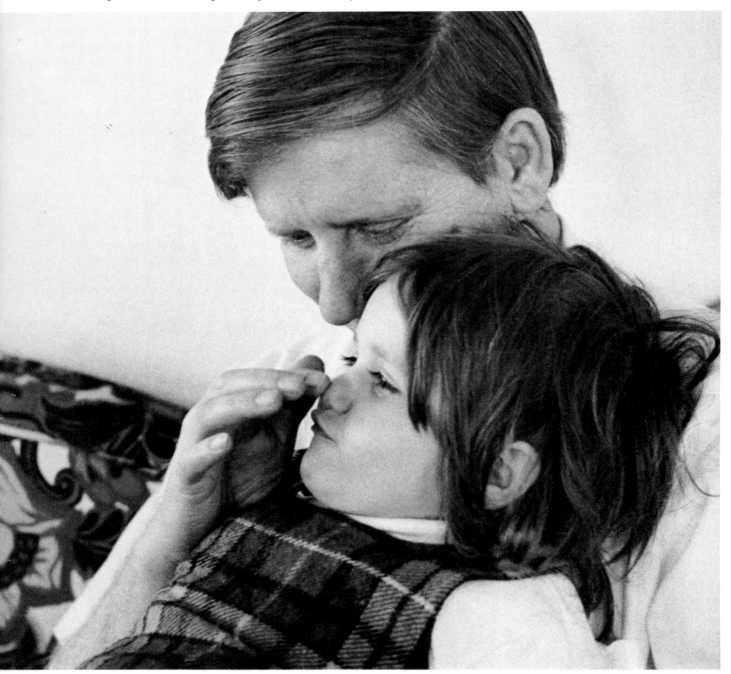

*Mary Ann, aged five, snuggles in her father's lap. The
children, born healthy and normal, have learned to communicate
with their father by following their mother's lead. They know
that "show daddy what you have" means placing it in his hands.*

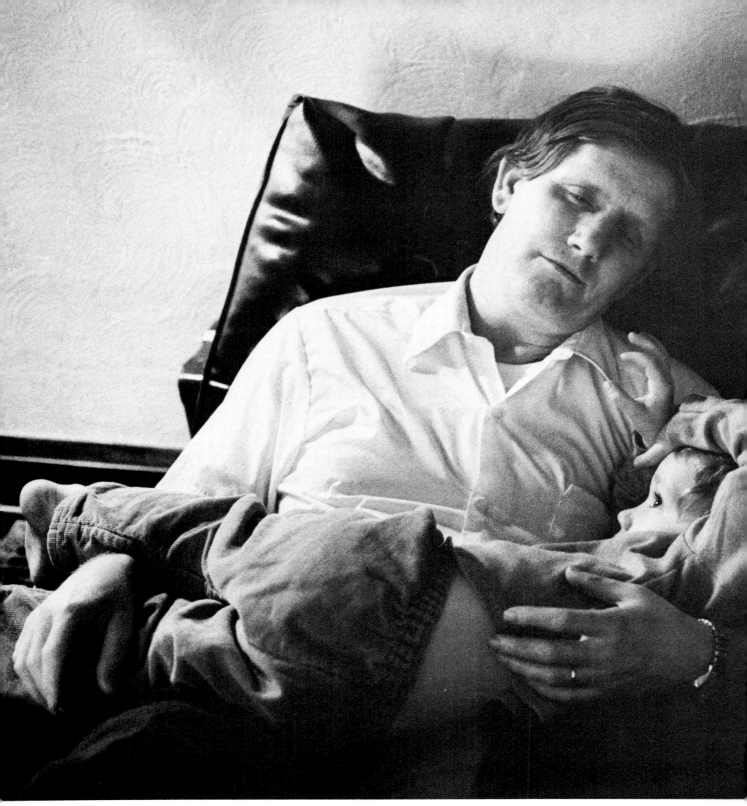

*Tired after a day in the office, Edwards relaxes in a comfortable
chair with Brian sprawled across his lap. The notion of seeing
his children's faces is to him only an abstraction: ''I have no need
to see the family,'' he said simply. ''I know all about them.''*

CHAPTER 5

Surgery under a microscope

Cataract removal—safe, sure and easy
Precision repairs with a laser
Draining the eye to save remnants of sight
A new age of ear surgery
Rebuilding the hearing mechanism
A 20-minute cure for deafness

When prizefighter Earnie Shavers battled Larry Holmes for the heavyweight title of the World Boxing Council in September 1979, the bout almost cost him dearly. He took a steady pounding from Holmes and lost the fight when the referee declared a technical knockout in the 11th round. At the time, he did not seem badly hurt, but later his left eye swelled shut. When the swelling subsided five days afterward, he discovered that his vision was badly blurred. A blow to Shavers' eye had ripped loose two thirds of the outer edge of his retina, the light-sensitive tissue at the back of the eye that transmits messages to the brain. The loose flap then folded over the rest of the retina.

Not long ago, such an extensive injury would certainly have spelled an abrupt end to Shavers' career and probably have doomed him to blindness in the injured eye. Instead, within two weeks after his championship fight, Earnie Shavers was on the operating table at Johns Hopkins University Hospital in Baltimore, his eye deadened to pain, while surgeons wielded a tiny cryoprobe, a freezing instrument, to bond the flap of the torn retina back in place. Less than five months later, his vision clear and his retina secure, Shavers returned to the ring.

Although the extent of Shavers' injury was unusual, his spectacular recovery was not. Miracles like this one are performed every day, not only on eyes, but also on ears, at hundreds of medical centers throughout the industrialized world. The repair of these essential organs is made possible by an armory of precision instruments that were developed after World War II. In addition to the retina-bonding cryoprobe, doctors routinely use the intense beams of light from lasers to destroy abnormal blood vessels growing on the retinas of diabetics, or to punch a hole in the iris to relieve the blinding pressure of glaucoma. Through an incision about an eighth of an inch long, they also bombard the eye with high-frequency sound waves to chop up a lens clouded by the opaque spots of cataracts.

In the ear, surgeons employ miniature scalpels to sculpt pieces of bone, cartilage and plastic into new pathways for sound. With electric drills tinier than a dentist's, they excavate infected tissue from behind the ear, or even bypass a damaged oval window—the tiny hole that opens into the inner ear—by drilling a new one.

But the one tool that has truly revolutionized eye and ear surgery is a sophisticated new version of an old device, the microscope. By bringing small, hidden parts of the body into view, the specialized operating microscope enables surgeons to rival the feats of craftsmen who engrave the Lord's Prayer on a dot smaller than the head of a pin. For example, the sutures that hold a corneal transplant in place are just one fourth as thick as a human hair.

Eye and ear surgery has been a very limited medical art for most of human history. Physicians have long known how to lance the eardrum to drain infection, and cataract removal, one of the most ancient of all surgical procedures, dates back at least 3,000 years. Early physicians believed that the lens, not the retina, was the center of vision and that

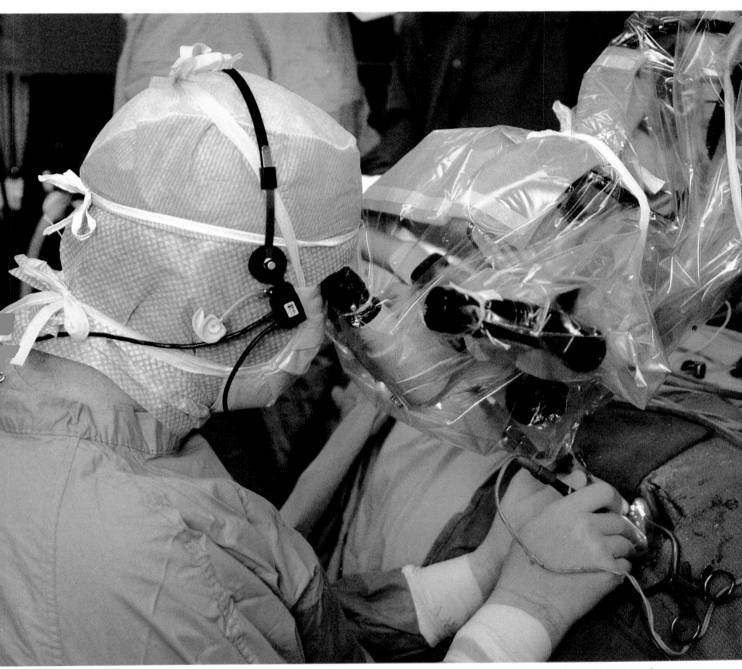

*His head swathed in a sterile mask, Los Angeles surgeon
William House watches his work with Lilliputian tools through a
plastic-wrapped microscope. He is drilling through bone
behind the ear to reach a pea-sized tumor that is lodged in the
inner ear and impairs balance. Next he will extract the growth,
using scissors and scalpels the size of an embroidery needle.*

the cataract was a membrane or a collection of corrupt "humors"—fluids—in front of the lens. Their remedy was to stick a long needle into the eye and push the lens back into the interior of the eye, supposedly away from the cataract. Sometimes this did indeed open a clear line of vision. More often, though, the opaque lens simply returned to its original site. Or the patient was blinded permanently because of infection or hemorrhage.

By the 19th Century, surgeons understood the steps needed to correct many eye and ear disorders. Without adequate lighting and magnification, or reliable means of controlling infection, surgery remained risky, to be sure. Nevertheless, history records some feats accomplished under difficult circumstances. In 1876, a German physician, Dr. Johann Kessel, attempted to restore a patient's hearing by opening the eardrum and operating on the stapes, or stirrup bone, just a tenth of an inch long, which had blocked sound when it became immobilized. Dr. Kessel performed the operation wearing only ordinary spectacles and working by the reflected light of an oil lamp. Obviously, the results of such surgery depended greatly on feel, guesswork—and luck.

In the early days of this century, electric lamps worn on head straps, hand-held magnifying lenses and special magnifying spectacles dispelled some of the guesswork. But these tools were awkward. The surgeon often ended up bending stiff-necked over the patient, straining to keep the operating field in focus.

The foundations of modern eye and ear surgery were laid in 1921, when a Swedish surgeon used a standard laboratory microscope while draining an infected ear. Over the next few decades, other ear surgeons improved on this basic tool, adding, for example, binocular lenses to provide the depth perception crucial for exacting surgery.

The breakthrough came in 1953, when the noted West German optical firm Carl Zeiss, Inc., produced a movable operating microscope that could be hung from the ceiling or mounted on a floor stand. It had variable magnification and a through-the-lens lighting system capable of casting shadowless illumination into the smallest confines of the human body. And unlike most microscopes, which jam their lenses close to the object under study, this new one was designed to leave ample working distance, giving surgeons room to maneuver their instruments and fingers.

Operations in a Lilliputian world

The human hand is capable of remarkably intricate maneuvers, so long as the eye can see what the hand is doing. But it takes long hours of training to gain the control needed for operating under the microscope, where the slightest movement may seem like a giant swipe. Painstakingly, the surgeon learns to work not with his wrists but with his fingers only, moving just a fraction of an inch at a time to manipulate a variety of scalpels, needles and probes—all scaled down to the Lilliputian world of the microscope. Perched on a stool, staring into the eyepieces, he appears strangely motionless. Only his fingers—and feet or chin, working the controls of the microscope—move ever so slightly.

The surgeon's task is simplified somewhat by microscopes that are increasingly elaborate and automatic. Today's models magnify up to 40 times. Most have extra sets of eyepieces for one or two assistants. With motorized foot pedals and chin switches, the surgeon can move the lens from side to side and front to back, adjust the magnification and focus, zoom in on the operating field, and activate instruments, all the while keeping his hands free.

Although microsurgery has fostered some questionable new practices—such as operations to correct nearsightedness (opposite)—it has vastly improved the precision and safety of a number of routine procedures. With the microscope, the surgeon can easily locate and extract foreign bodies from the ear canal and the cornea of the eye. Powerful magnification makes it possible to sew up incisions with greater accuracy —using needles the thickness of two red blood cells—and thus avoid leakage or too much tension. The incisions heal faster, with less pain, inflammation and scar tissue.

Most significant, though, are the new frontiers opened up to surgeons through the lenses of the microscope. Thanks to microsurgery, daring rescues from the isolation of blindness and deafness have become routine. High magnification reduces the risks of working close to the delicate sensory links with the brain—the retina and optic nerve in the eye and the cochlea and acoustic nerve in the ear—where a surgical misstep can cause irreparable nerve damage and permanent loss of sight or hearing. Skilled treatment of the other parts of the organs is equally crucial, because it determines whether sound or light will ever reach the delicate receptors that transmit messages to the brain.

A simple look at the anatomy of these organs explains why eye surgery came thousands of years before ear operations and is still the more prevalent. The eye, filled with transparent structures and fluids from front to back, is a remarkably accessible organ, amenable to extensive sorts of repairs that would be impractical in the ear. Even the retina, which, like the inner ear, is an extension of the brain, holds no secrets. The doctor can look at it directly from outside the eye. He can send dye through its veins and examine its blood supply, bombard it with laser beams aimed through the pupil, and freeze spots on it from behind to seal holes or tears. And by doing a vitrectomy—removing the fluid, or vitreous humor, that fills the space between lens and retina—he can work directly on the retina.

Cataract removal—safe, sure and easy

Even the removal of cataracts—within easy reach of ancient surgeons—has been revolutionized. In recent years, microsurgery, extreme cold, high-frequency sound waves, and jet-age plastics have combined to make a cataract operation one of the safest and most successful of all surgical procedures. Just a few decades ago, a patient whose cornea had been cut to remove a cataract-clouded lens was forced to remain in the hospital for two weeks after surgery, his head immobilized with sandbags to keep the loosely stitched wound still while it healed. Today, the wound is closed with microscopic stitches, and a cataract patient is up and walking around two or three hours after surgery. He might even go home from the hospital the same day.

The basic steps in removing cataracts were developed in the mid-1700s by a French surgeon, Dr. Jacques Daviel, who discovered that removing the clouded part of the lens pro-

A fine scalpel slices a patient's anesthetized cornea (upper picture, below) in a controversial treatment for nearsightedness that can eliminate the need for eyeglasses. The eight cuts, radiating like spokes (lower photo), flatten the cornea, reducing its curve and sharpening focus. Though often effective, the operation risks permanent damage to tissues.

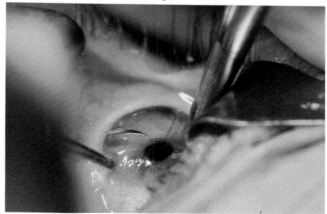

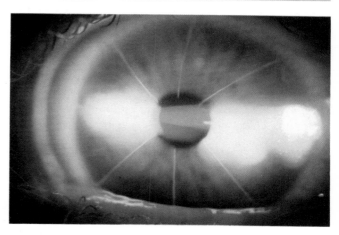

duced better results than pushing the lens back into the eye. Using instruments of his own design, Dr. Daviel made an incision at the edge of the cornea, cut through the capsule of the lens with a sharp needle, and then scooped out the lens contents with a spoonlike device. But in some cases he found it difficult to remove all the lens contents, and often the eye became inflamed.

Today, surgeons avoid these problems in either of two ways. Most often they remove the entire lens capsule with the aid of a cryoprobe, a rod whose tip can be cooled to −40° F. by refrigerant gas flowing inside it. When touched to the lens, the cryoprobe freezes fast to it, just as an ice-cube tray sticks to wet fingers. With this firm grasp, the surgeon easily lifts the lens out of the eye. The technique, developed in 1960, is successful 98 per cent of the time.

Microsurgery and mechanized irrigation and suction devices have also improved Dr. Daviel's original method, making it possible to leave part of the capsule in the eye, as he did, while thoroughly removing all other lens material. An ultrasonic needle, vibrating with inaudibly high-pitched sound waves, is inserted through an incision in the capsule. The rapid vibrations of the needle pulverize the lens contents into minute particles that can be sucked out through another hollow needle. The tiny incision is closed with just a few stitches and is virtually rupture-proof.

The most dramatic advance in cataract treatment attacks a problem that is created by the surgery itself. When the clouded lens is partially or entirely removed, light can once again reach the retina; but without the focusing material of the lens, the image is badly blurred. Until recently only a partial remedy was available: thick spectacles that clear up some of the blur. Today a new lens can be implanted in the eye to replace the cataract-stricken one that was removed.

The notion of lens implants is not new. Casanova, the Venetian adventurer of the 18th Century, referred to attempts at such surgery in his memoirs. But the first successful operation was not performed until 1949, when a London ophthalmologist, Dr. Harold Ridley, fashioned an artificial lens from the clear plastic used for the canopies of British warplanes. This material had been well tested in the eyes of injured World War II pilots, many of whom had been struck by bits of flying plastic when their planes were hit by enemy gunfire. The plastic proved to be inert; it caused virtually no inflammation even after it had remained embedded in some of the pilots' eyes nine years after injury. Today, lens implants are made of this plastic or, in some cases, of a section sliced from a human cornea and shaped on a small lathe *(page 132)*. The substitute is slipped into position behind the iris or in front of it.

Even when a replacement lens is implanted, cataract surgery takes only about an hour and can be done under local anesthesia. As long as the patient is in good general health, age is no obstacle to the sight-restoring procedure. In 1981, a New York City man had cataracts removed and artificial

An artificial cornea in a nut and a bolt

The bits of plastic hardware at right form a valuable addition to the arsenal of the eye surgeon. When a cornea, the eye's transparent covering, is irreparably damaged and a corneal transplant *(page 132)* fails, these replacement parts can restore 20/20 vision.

The main component, a mushroom-shaped bolt that serves as both cornea and lens, is anchored inside the eyeball by a white nut. Joining the two pieces is a delicate job. A hole is drilled into the eye for the bolt; a separate incision is made for the nut, which is slid to a position behind the hole. Finally the bolt, held in a suction cup, is screwed into the nut to fit snugly against the eye's outer curve.

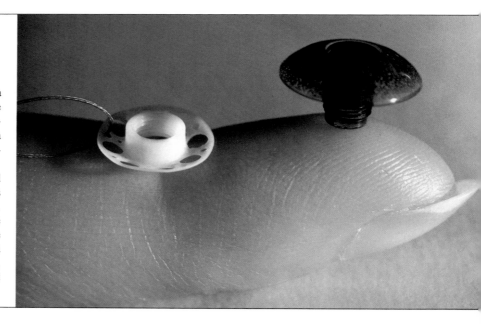

lenses implanted in both eyes when he was 100 years old. Asked why he chose to undergo two operations at this stage of life, he replied: ''I wanted to really be able to see the beauty of the day.''

Precision repairs with a laser

The revolution that microsurgical tools have brought in the treatment of common eye ailments such as cataracts has been paralleled for rarer disorders that, in the past, generally ended in blindness. One new instrument, the laser, which generates an intense, sharply focused beam of light, can painlessly burn precise holes in tissue in a fraction of a second to remedy several eye disorders. It has proved valuable for treating closed-angle glaucoma, in which a defect in the iris, by keeping the eye's natural fluid from reaching channels that would normally drain it out of the eye, causes pressure to increase inside the eyeball. In the early stages of the disease, surgeons can relieve pressure within the eye by making a small incision or taking a snip out of the iris so that the fluid can drain. This operation is quite simple, but the laser offers an even simpler alternative—one that requires no hospitalization and none of the emotional ordeal of operating-room surgery.

The patient, sitting up, places his chin on a special rest to keep his head steady. After using a drop or two of anesthetic to numb the cornea, the ophthalmologist places a contact lens on the eye to help him focus the laser beam on the iris. Quickly, he taps a foot pedal four or five times. With each flash, lasting just $^2/_{10}$ second, the laser burns a little deeper into the iris, eventually making a microscopic hole. Trapped fluid immediately seeps out, reducing pressure to halt the progress of glaucoma. The procedure takes only 15 minutes, and in many cases the patient is able to go home immediately afterward. A 1980 survey of 600 patients who received this laser treatment at Johns Hopkins Hospital, in Baltimore, found the technique successful in 96 of 100 cases.

The laser has had its greatest impact, however, on treatment of diabetic retinopathy, in which abnormal blood vessels and scar tissue spread over the retina to obscure vision. Only the destruction of the abnormal tissues can prevent blindness. As early as 1949, ophthalmologists attempted to burn the tissues away with beams of sunlight focused through a complicated optical system. Later, various other powerful

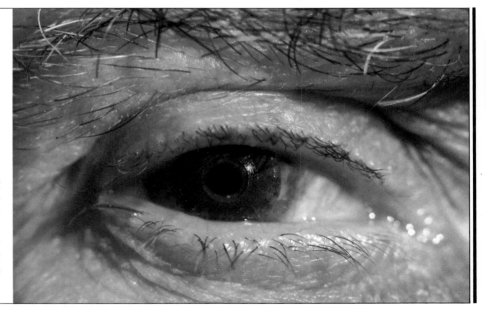

In the two-part artificial cornea at left, the domed bolt head provides color and support; a lens built into its threaded shaft focuses light upon the retina, and the entire shaft screws into the white nut, which is implanted inside the eyeball. The bluish surgical thread attached to the nut is a safety device used to retrieve the piece if it drifts down into the eye during surgery.

Implanted and secured, the artificial cornea looks astonishingly natural; the color of the bolt head is chosen to match the patient's iris. Unlike a natural iris, however, the bolt shaft cannot widen and narrow in response to weak and strong light; a patient must adapt to extremes by using extra light or wearing dark glasses.

light sources were used for this so-called photocoagulation, but no other instrument can match the laser for the intensity and precision of its beam.

The laser treatment does not affect the outer eye. The physician uses drops to widen the pupil, then aims the beam through the open pupil directly at the retina. The beam passes through the transparent cornea without heating the tissue, much as sunlight passes through a clear window without heating the glass. With rapid taps on the foot-pedal control, the doctor peppers the retina with short bursts of light, producing as many as 1,500 burns in each eye. To minimize the strain on the patient, treatment is often spread over several sessions lasting about 45 minutes each. Even without a local anesthetic, the patient feels only a slight irritation and perhaps a headache.

The intense bursts of light from the laser do more than seal off abnormal blood vessels. They also apparently destroy the stimulus that causes such vessels to grow. The ones that are there simply wither away. Best of all, they rarely grow back.

Laser photocoagulation cannot be used if broken blood vessels have been causing persistent bleeding into the vitreous humor, because the bloody vitreous would prevent the doctor from seeing where to focus the beam. Photocoagulation also is of little help for patients whose vision is already severely impaired. In such cases, the last hope is vitrectomy, in which the vitreous humor is removed to give the surgeon a clear view inside the eyeball. It can be not only a necessary preliminary to photocoagulation but also a valuable technique for repairing severe retinal tears, treating injuries to the eye, removing mysterious membranes that sometimes start growing on the retina, and extracting lens material left in the eye after cataract surgery.

Draining the eye to save remnants of sight

Not many years ago, the loss of vitreous was something to be feared, since changes in this gelatinous material could cause serious complications. The vitreous is somewhat like egg white, a gel containing fibrous bands. If those bands get caught up in a wound, for example, they can pull on the retina and tear it loose.

In 1970 a technique for safely removing the vitreous fluid without disturbing the front of the eye and without damaging the back was developed at the University of Miami by Dr. Robert Machemer. Working with an engineer, Jean-Marie Parel, Dr. Machemer designed an instrument known as the Vitreous Infusion Suction Cutter—VISC for short. This ingenious device, which looks something like a large fountain pen with a needle on the end, simultaneously cuts through the vitreous, sucks it out through a tube and replaces it with a special saline solution.

In spite of the potential benefits of vitrectomy, the procedure is considered a hazardous one—"high-stakes surgery," was the way it was characterized recently by Dr. Ronald G. Michels of Johns Hopkins. It has the highest rate of complications of any eye operation, partly because the surgeon is operating close to or directly on the retina and partly because the eyes on which it is performed are already in a precarious condition. It is the treatment of last resort, even for diabetic retinopathy. If there is hemorrhaging into the vitreous, for example, most doctors prefer to delay for six months to a year before undertaking the operation, to see if the eye will clear up on its own.

Those were the risks weighed not long ago by Dr. Michels and a patient who, diabetic for 24 of his 25 years, had developed severe diabetic retinopathy. Photocoagulation, done perhaps too late, did not help, and before long he was legally blind. Scar tissue had already pulled loose the retina of his left eye. Normally, that eye would have been operated on first. But the patient decided to take a chance on repairing his "good" eye first, in hopes that his vision would be improved enough to let him return to work.

Just before surgery, the patient's eyelashes were clipped, and he received several applications of eye drops to dilate his pupil—essential if the surgeon was to have a clear view of the interior of the eye. When Dr. Michels entered the room, the patient was already anesthetized and draped. A surgical assistant squeezed additional drops on the patient's eye to keep the pupil dilated. She then made a tiny incision in the skin at each corner of the eye, so the lids could be opened wider, and fastened the lids open with a metal device called a

Muscles snipped and stretched to curb an errant eye

The eyes of the child pictured here are her most striking feature—but their beauty was marred, from infancy, by the inward drift of the left one. Jenny Monroe's condition, convergent strabismus, made her "cross-eyed," in the blunt language of playmates.

But strabismus affects far more than appearance, for when malfunctioning muscles allow the eyes to point in different directions *(below)* the eyes perceive two unmatched versions of an object and send a double image to the brain. To resolve this confusion, the brain may tune out the image from one eye, and in time lose its use completely.

Jenny's left eye was partially straightened by thick lenses she wore from the age of three to correct another problem—farsightedness *(see page 83)*, a focusing disorder, which often goes hand in hand with strabismus. As she grew older, though, the glasses became less effective in controlling the drift of her eye. Her doctor finally decided on surgery.

The operation is relatively simple. It readjusts the pulling power of the two muscles that anchor the misdirected eye at either side: One muscle is tightened and the other is loosened, thus bringing that eye into normal alignment.

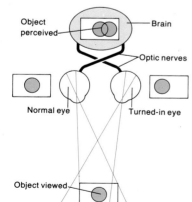
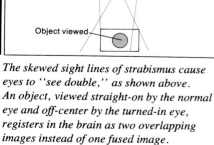

The skewed sight lines of strabismus cause eyes to "see double," as shown above. An object, viewed straight-on by the normal eye and off-center by the turned-in eye, registers in the brain as two overlapping images instead of one fused image.

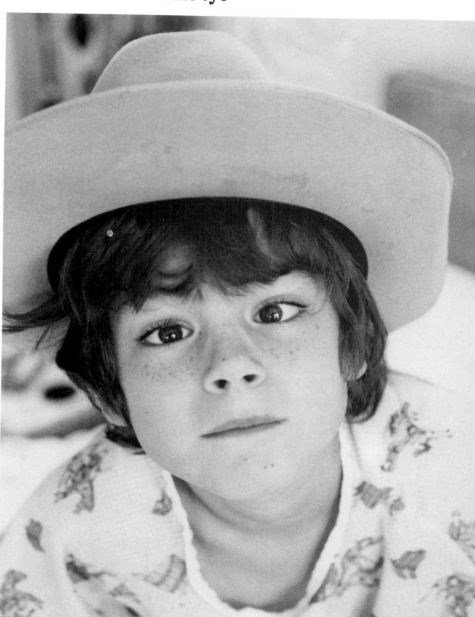

Awaiting surgery, seven-year-old Jenny Monroe plays in a pediatric ward, wearing a bright hospital gown and her father's hat. The pronounced drift of the left eye kept her eyes from working together to perceive a normal, three-dimensional image. Her parents feared she would so favor the view from one eye that vision from the other would atrophy through disuse.

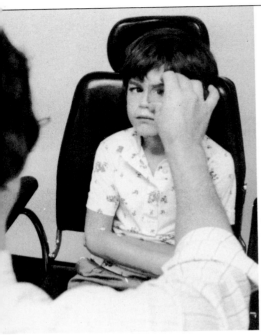

During a preoperative examination, a clinic doctor measures the angle of Jenny's deviant eye with a prism, to determine how much correction she needs. Later, the patient had some jitters: "If anything came out wrong, could I be blind?" she asked. Her doctor, Robert Petersen, assured her that that could not happen.

Jenny arrives at the hospital the day before her operation—"sort of excited and sort of scared" —toting suitcase, stuffed animals and gifts from her parents. Her mother remained in Jenny's hospital room throughout her two-night stay.

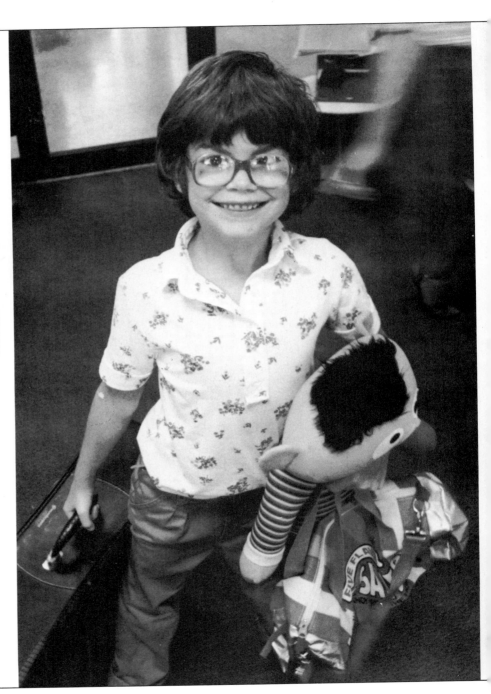

The operation under way, Jenny's left eye is isolated by sterile drapings and held open with a lid-spreading tool; Dr. Petersen lifts a pared-away muscle with a surgical hook as he prepares to change its position on the eyeball. The scissor-like clamps hold black threads that are sewn to the eye and used to pull it around during surgery. The threads will be removed at the end.

Two muscles (red) are cut (left), then reattached (right) to align an eye. First the surgeon moves the medial rectus farther back (black bar), loosening it. Then he shortens the lateral rectus and resews it to its original attachment, to pull the eye straight.

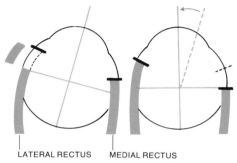

LATERAL RECTUS   MEDIAL RECTUS

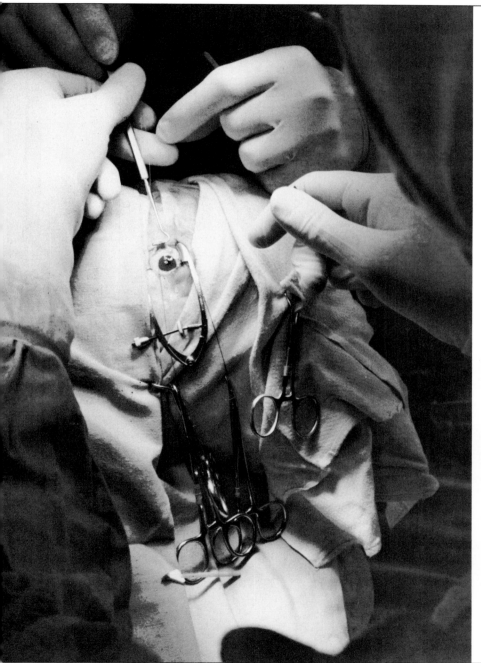

Dr. Petersen tests Jenny's eyes several days after the operation with the Worth Four-Dot Test. While Jenny wears a red lens over one eye and a green lens over the other, he shines a flashlight displaying one red, one white and two green dots. Normal vision sees one red dot (with the red-filtered eye), two green dots (with the other eye), and the white dot (through the fusion of both filtered eyes). Jenny passed.

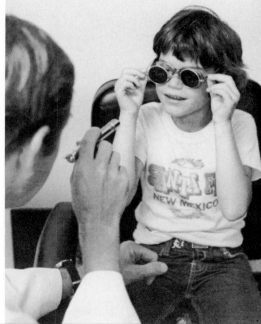

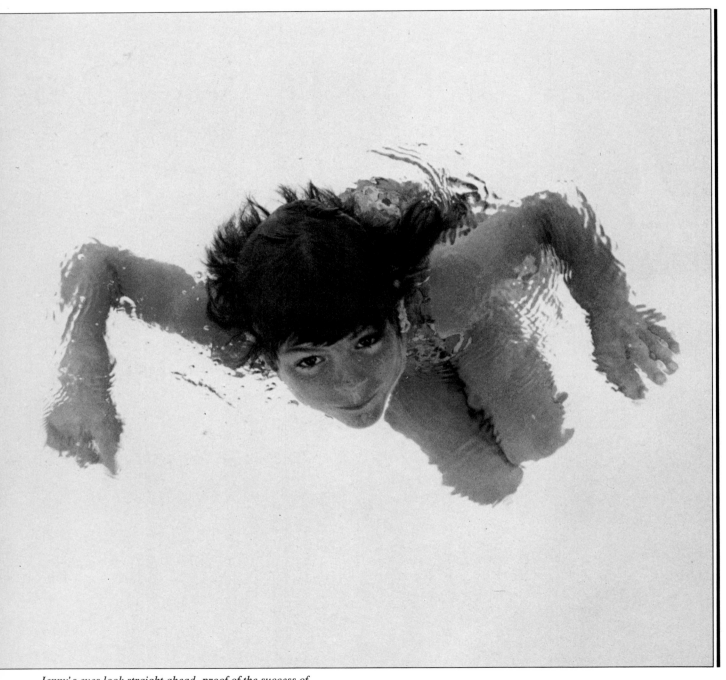

Jenny's eyes look straight ahead, proof of the success of surgery, as she splashes in her family's backyard pool following a month-long ban. Swimming was the only thing she could not do after the operation, because of the risk of infection.

speculum. As she worked, a nurse squirted fluid on the cornea every few minutes to keep it moist.

The operating microscope was brought into position above the patient, and Dr. Michels was ready to begin. Peering into the lens, he carefully snipped open the transparent conjunctival membrane covering the eye and folded it back, to expose the surface of the sclera, or white of the eye. Next, he made three tiny incisions in different parts of the sclera. Instead of the single VISC, Dr. Michels prefers to use three separate vitrectomy instruments, which he feels give him greater flexibility. Through one incision, the surgical assistant inserted a tube that would inject a saline solution to keep the eye from collapsing when its vitreous fluid was removed. With a few stitches in the white of the eye, she secured the tube. In the second opening, Dr. Michels inserted a fiber-optic tube, containing fine glass fibers that pipe light into the work area. Into the third hole went the cutting-suction tool, which he controlled with his right hand while his left aimed the light tube. The assistant placed a contact lens on the patient's eye to compensate for the curvature of the cornea and enable the microscope to focus on the back of the eye.

Dr. Michels kicked off his shoes and positioned his feet on the floor pedals that controlled the microscope and mechanized instruments. ''Vitreous surgery is like driving a Volkswagen,'' he commented. ''You need both hands and both feet.'' Then, a call of ''Lights out!'' and the room was plunged into darkness except for the light from the microscope and the tube inside the patient's eye.

Viewed through the microscope, the cutting-suction device, magnified 10 times, moved slowly and deliberately under the steady guidance of the surgeon's fingers. Powered by compressed air, its guillotine-like blade chopped through the gel and stringy bands of the vitreous. Simultaneously, through a hollow tube above the blade, the probe sucked out gel, bits of tissue and a small amount of blood. In this delicately balanced system, the exact volume removed was immediately replaced with saline solution piped through the infusion tube on the other side of the eye.

As the probe approached the retina, the full destructive nature of diabetic retinopathy became grimly obvious. A normal retina is smooth, its delicate network of blood vessels as clearly visible as the lines on a road map. The macula, where sharp vision is centered, shows up as a vaguely defined yellowish area, the optic nerve as a distinct yellow circle. In this patient's eye, the scene was different. Blood vessels and white chunks of scar tissue dangled from the retina, jutting out into the vitreous. The macula and optic nerve were virtually obscured by the debris. Scattered throughout the diseased retina were hundreds of gray dots, the remnants of previous efforts to repair it with laser burns.

If the patient was to see again, Dr. Michels had to remove as much of the diseased tissue as possible without harming the retina. Withdrawing the cutting probe, he called for a succession of specialized instruments: a probe with tiny electrodes to seal off the abnormal blood vessels with electric current, a pick to dissect bits of scar tissue, miniature scissors to snip membranes more firmly attached to the retina and to cut through tissue that could not safely be attacked with the cutting probe, a hollow vacuum needle to suck up the debris.

During these delicate maneuvers, the operating room was hushed. Only the beep-beep of the device monitoring the patient's pulse and the quiet strains of music from a ceiling speaker broke the silence. As Dr. Michels approached the macula, he said softly: ''This is where my heart beats faster. We have here a young man, and we're operating on his better eye. What he sees for the rest of his life depends on what happens right now.''

At last satisfied that he had cleaned away all the damage he could, Dr. Michels made a final scan of the inside of the eye. A few shreds of tissue still clung around the optic nerve, which, as the blind spot of the eye, was unhindered by their presence. The vitrectomy instruments were withdrawn and plugs inserted in the incisions to keep any fluid from leaking out. Then, using a hand-held lens and ophthalmoscope, Dr. Michels again examined the retina from outside the eye to make sure there had been no accidental damage.

All was well. Dr. Michels removed the plugs and stitched up the incisions. The conjunctiva was edged back into place and sutured, as were the incisions at the corners of the eye. The surgical assistant injected an antibiotic into the eye,

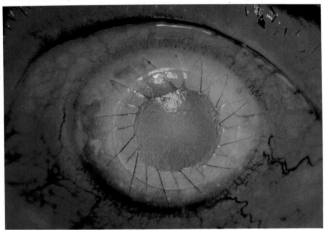

This eye has received a new cornea: The patient's diseased cornea was cut away and a healthy cornea was stitched in its place, the sutures appearing as a star-shaped outline. During recovery the cornea will be stained every day with a greenish-yellow dye that adheres to abrasions but washes away from normal tissue; when no stain adheres at all, healing is complete.

removed the lid fastener, and rubbed some cream on the lids to keep them from sticking together. The eye was patched and a protective shield placed over it.

As the patient was wheeled from the operating room, Dr. Michels relaxed and smiled. A long day of surgery had gotten off to a happy start. He had been able to remove the abnormal tissue without damaging the retina. Without the strands of vitreous gel to serve as scaffolding, the tissue and blood vessels would not grow back. The patient would remain in the hospital about five days. The patch would stay on for a week. After that, the patient could resume normal eye activity, although he would have to avoid strenuous work for several weeks. "This young man's vision will never be completely normal, because advanced retinopathy causes some permanent damage," Dr. Michels said. "But he might well be able to drive again and possibly even read." In an hour and a half of incredibly delicate eyeball cleaning, sight was restored to an eye that had been blind.

A new age of ear surgery

The tools and techniques that have made possible intricate repairs to the eye have had an even greater impact on treatment of the ear. Its working parts are so minute and so hidden that not until the time of World War II could operations be performed safely and reliably on the hearing mechanism.

Unlike the easy-to-reach eye, the delicate parts of the ear are surrounded by a fortress of cartilage, flesh and bone, sealed off behind a taut membrane at the end of a narrow tunnel. The inner ear—counterpart of the eye's retina—is deep within the skull, next to the brain, and remains somewhat mysterious. When hearing is lost because of damage to its nerves or other fragile parts, doctors still can do little.

The great advances of the past decades, which have restored hearing to thousands of people, have centered on the middle ear and the mastoid area just behind it. Thanks to microsurgery, the eardrum, which conveys sound from air into the ear mechanism, can be reconstructed; the three minuscule bones of the middle ear, which transmit vibrations to the inner ear, can be repaired or replaced; and the bony air pockets filling the mastoid cavity can be cleared of diseased bone and tissue that hinder repair efforts by spreading infection to the ear.

The outer ear, of course, has always been accessible to physicians. This open pathway permits one ear operation that has been in wide use for more than a century: a myringotomy, in which the doctor uses a sharp, pointed knife to lance a swollen eardrum and release infected fluid trapped behind it. The earache, one of childhood's commonest ailments, often results when respiratory infections reach the ear through the Eustachian tubes; the infection stimulates the ear to produce defensive fluids, which clog the Eustachian tubes so that they can no longer serve for drainage. Fluid builds up in the middle ear, pressing painfully on the eardrum. The small slit of the myringotomy provides a temporary drain and brings quick relief, then soon heals shut. A baby who has cried all night from the pain of an infected ear generally falls into a peaceful sleep minutes after the swollen eardrum is pierced.

The simple myringotomy for infection is much less common now than it was as recently as the 1950s. It has been made largely obsolete by antibiotics. Drugs such as penicillin quickly cure the infection and the earache. But even after the infection disappears, excess fluid may remain. This "fluid ear" is treated by a variation of the myringotomy. The surgeon, with the help of the operating microscope, punctures the eardrum but deliberately makes the hole stay open for some time, inserting a small plastic or stainless-steel tube to let air enter the middle ear. This new vent releases the vacuum that is created by the pressure of trapped fluid and allows it to escape down the Eustachian tube, much as a second hole punched in a soft-drink can will help the contents flow out more easily. Within six months, the fluid generally disappears and the inserted tube falls out of its own accord.

No earache can ever be ignored—not only because of the pain, but also because, if untreated, it can lead to serious, irreparable harm. The infection can spread to the mastoid region and inner ear, even threatening the brain. And within the middle ear, infection can leave permanent damage to the sound-transmitting mechanism.

Indeed, the middle-ear deterioration induced by chronic infection is one of the most common reasons for ear surgery among adults. Typically, the patient goes to the doctor complaining of hearing loss and a discharge from the ear. An examination reveals that persistent infection has worn a permanent hole in the eardrum and pus is draining into the external ear canal. If the patient hears reasonably well when a tuning fork or an electrical vibrator is held to the skull, but cannot hear well through the ear, damage to nerves of the inner ear can be ruled out, and the trouble lies in the middle ear, where it usually can be fixed.

The first step is to eliminate all traces of disease, so that there will be no source of recurring infection to undo the repairs to come. This may mean removal of infected bone and tissue from the mastoid region—a mastoidectomy—or from the middle-ear cavity itself.

Once the ear and mastoid are free of disease, the surgeon can concentrate on the repair work. In many cases, he must replace an eardrum that has been torn or eaten away and reconstruct bones that are partially or completely destroyed. The defect most often found is a gap in the sound-carrying chain of bones: hammer to anvil to stirrup. The long thin part of the anvil that meets the stirrup is generally the first to die and disintegrate, because its blood supply is limited. Sometimes the footplate of the stirrup becomes fixed in the oval window of the inner ear so that it can no longer transmit

sound vibrations. "One of the things about ear surgery is that you can never be exactly sure what you have to do until you get in there," recently remarked Dr. Hugh de Fries of Georgetown University. "It's like opening Pandora's box. You always have a surprise."

Rebuilding the hearing mechanism

To restore hearing by reconstructing the middle ear, many surgeons today prefer to operate in stages, fixing one part, then waiting for the patient to recover before working on the next defect some months later. This was the scheme followed at the Washington Hospital Center by Dr. de Fries and his associates in the case of a 26-year-old woman, a victim of chronic ear infection, who was suffering some hearing loss when she sought their help. First, a mastoidectomy cleared the area of infected tissue and bone. Next, the patient's eardrum, badly damaged by years of disease, was reconstructed. A final operation was needed a few months later to rebuild bones in her middle ear. Only then, two years after the beginning of treatment, could she recover her hearing.

For the first of the three operations, the mastoidectomy, some 200 surgical instruments of varying sizes had to be in readiness, although only a few dozen actually were used. The larger ones, designed for the outer ear and mastoid area, were arranged on the left side of a sterile table. The microsurgery instruments sat in their own numbered racks on the right side. A supply of tiny cotton balls, each smaller than the tip of a little finger, was carefully counted to assure that one would not unintentionally be left in the patient. There was no need to count the instruments. As small as they appeared to the naked eye, none could possibly get lost in the ear. Dominating the scene was the operating microscope, a huge motionless mechanical spider hanging from its ceiling mount, eyepieces jutting out like legs at odd angles.

After the patient was anesthetized and "prepped" for the operation, Dr. de Fries and his assistant, gowned and gloved, went to work. Using a scalpel and surgical instruments called dissectors, the surgeons made an incision behind the woman's ear and peeled back the skin and connective tissue overlying the bump of the mastoid bone, about three fourths of an inch from the ear. Then, with a burr-tipped drill like the one dentists use, Dr. de Fries cut a hole through the skull to expose the infection's haven—hundreds of tiny air pockets, connected to the middle ear by a corridor hidden about three quarters of an inch below the surface. This corridor was the surgeons' first target, for clearing it would give them a clear view of the boundaries their drill had to follow to avoid damaging vital surrounding structures: the facial nerve, the semicircular canals of the balance organ, a vein carrying

blood away from the brain, and the edge of the brain itself.

About halfway in toward the middle-ear connection, the doctors stopped, changed to smaller burrs for the drill, and began to use the microscope to guide their work as they inched closer to delicate nerve centers. Taking care to leave a thin shell of bone between the mastoid cavity and these crucial areas, Dr. de Fries moved the drill around the remaining air pockets in the mastoid, scouring out long-entrenched bits of infected bone and tissue.

A drain that restores an astronaut's balance

The most famous victim of Ménière's disease, an ear disorder that disturbs balance and hearing, was astronaut Alan B. Shepard Jr. *(below, right)*. After he made the first American flight into space, he was grounded by unpredictable attacks of vertigo—until a new operation *(below)* helped him so much that he was able to command the Apollo 14 moon landing in 1971.

Ménière's disease is surprisingly common, affecting as many as seven million Americans. The attacks are caused by an excess of the fluid that fills two interconnected organs of the inner ear—the cochlea, which translates sound-caused pressure changes in the

fluid into nerve signals, and the semicircular canals, which gauge movements of the fluid to control balance. The excess arises from unknown causes. In the cochlea, it diminishes hearing and sets off ringing noises, while in the semicircular canals it can so confuse balance that victims fall down.

Most sufferers are treated with drugs that regulate nerve impulses, stimulate circulation or limit bodily fluid levels. If drugs do not help, surgery can drain the excess fluid. The surgery is tricky because it is so close to the brain, but it relieves otherwise incurable vertigo and improves hearing in at least half the patients.

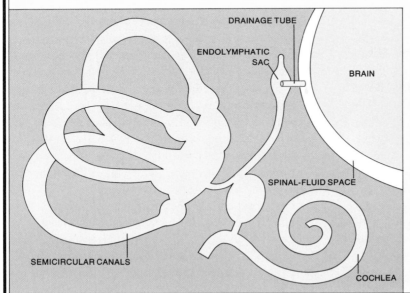

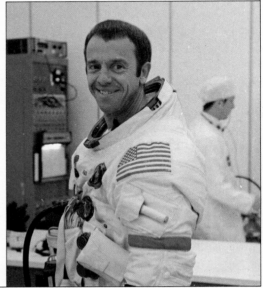

In an operation to relieve the dizziness and hearing loss of Ménière's disease, the surgeon installs a rubber tube linking the endolymphatic sac of the inner ear to the spinal-fluid space cushioning the brain. Into this brain cushion, the tube diverts the cause of the symptoms: an excess of the endolymph, which is fluid that fills the sac, the semicircular canals and the cochlea.

Suited up to fly once more, astronaut Alan B. Shepard Jr. prepares for a test before his 1971 trip to the moon. Grounded eight years earlier by the vertigo of Ménière's disease, he owed his comeback to the shunt operation diagrammed at left.

With the mastoid cleared, Dr. de Fries next turned to the connecting passage and, using even smaller drill tips, he cleaned out infected tissue from the middle ear. To provide more room for his work, Dr. de Fries at this point also removed the anvil bone, which lay detached from the stirrup and therefore was useless in passing along sound waves. Preserved in alcohol, it would later be used to rebuild a sound pathway through the middle ear.

Satisfied that the infected tissue had been cleaned out, the surgeons replaced the flaps of skin and connective tissue over the hollowed-out mastoid space behind the ear, and sewed up the incision. In place of disease-riddled cubbyholes, the mastoid was now one large air cell that opened into the patient's middle ear and permitted the free circulation of air necessary to keep infection at bay. But the drying-out and healing process would be a long one. Thirteen months elapsed before doctors were ready to reenter the woman's ear for the second stage—fashioning a new eardrum to replace the one that had been destroyed by infection.

The second operation was performed by Dr. Ziad Deeb, Director of Otolaryngology at the center. As soon as the patient was anesthetized and prepared for surgery, as before, Dr. Deeb's assistant pulled the microscope into position above the table and adjusted his view of the ear canal. While Dr. Deeb watched through the second eyepiece, the assistant inserted a tiny scalpel into the ear and made an incision on the wall of the ear canal about one half inch from the eardrum. This would give him access for later examination of the middle ear. Pushing the microscope aside, the assistant then made a thin incision behind the ear, tracing the line of the mastoidectomy scar.

Extending the incision, Dr. Deeb snipped connective tissue that he would use as material for a new eardrum. In the past whole skin was employed for this purpose, but hair follicles and other skin cells often gave rise to unwanted growths in the middle ear. Connective tissue, lacking these extra cells, has proved to be the ideal graft. Placed across a perforated eardrum membrane, it serves as a bridge on which new skin can grow from the ear canal and build a new eardrum. The graft itself eventually dissolves.

Dr. Deeb was now ready to approach the eardrum and middle ear. He pulled the microscope into position, and the room lights were dimmed. The illumination from the microscope alone provided the clearest view. With forceps, he gently pulled the tattered eardrum membrane out of the rim in which it sat. Almost all of the membrane itself had been eroded away by infection, but the remaining rim would give the graft a foundation.

With the eardrum lifted away, the middle ear came into view as a whitish cavity. Gingerly, Dr. Deeb probed with a tiny pick, surveying the site of the previous operation. Fortunately, the area had remained clear of infection since the first surgery, and Dr. Deeb could easily assess the damage to the two bones still in place: the hammer, or malleus, and the stirrup, or stapes. "There's the handle of the malleus," he reported, "and down here is the stapes. See it move! It's not fixed, which means that we won't have to replace the stapes after all." The anvil, of course, was still safe in a jar on the shelf. It was not reinserted at this point—for several reasons. Any bone reconstruction done now would be covered only by the graft, not by a secure eardrum, so the whole arrangement would be quite unstable. And there was always the chance that the graft would not take, and that an infection would develop and undo the repairs.

The immediate task, then, was to seal off the middle ear behind a new eardrum. Dr. Deeb packed the entire middle-ear cavity with pieces of gelfoam—a porous, cushiony material made from gelatin. He then laid the graft on top of the gelfoam. Additional squares of gelfoam were placed along the outer edges of the graft to help sandwich it in place until it healed. No sutures were needed. Within about a month, the gelfoam would be absorbed into the patient's tissues, leaving the graft firmly attached to the ear-canal wall. New skin would grow in from either side of the graft to form a completely new eardrum.

Two hours and 15 minutes after they had made the first incision, the surgeons placed a final dressing over the ear. The patient, when she awoke, would feel little pain. If no complications developed, she would go home the following day. With a clean, dry middle ear and a new eardrum, the woman now had two thirds of the equipment for a healthy, functioning ear.

In the final crucial step, doctors once again would have to enter the woman's middle ear, to reinsert her anvil in a rebuilt chain of bones capable of carrying sound waves from the eardrum to the oval window. This new pathway, at last, would enable her to hear normally again.

In this case, the anvil—the middle bone—had been removed to facilitate the cleaning of the middle ear. It and the other two were in satisfactory condition, and after the first two stages of surgery were past, the anvil could be put back in place to restore sound transmission. In other cases, any of the three may be damaged, either by infection or by deterioration from other causes. Each bone is essential—the hammer to pick up vibrations from the eardrum and pass them to the anvil, the anvil to transfer them from hammer to stirrup, and the stirrup to transfer them through the oval window to the fluid inside the cochlea. When the surgeon repairing the middle ear gets inside, he may find any of these tiny, vital bones misshapen or frozen rigidly to its neighboring surface.

One of the most common types of middle-ear repair sets free a stirrup that has become immobilized because a disease—otosclerosis—has caused a new growth of bone around it. The pioneering 19th Century ear surgeon Dr. Johann Kessel had the right idea in trying to restore hearing in otosclerosis by freeing an immobile stirrup, but without antibiotics or adequate lighting and magnification, he and other surgeons who tried similar techniques failed more often than they succeeded.

A 20-minute cure for deafness

Finally, in the mid-1950s, doctors developed a 20-minute operation, known as a stapedectomy, that has since rescued many thousands of people from deafness of varying degrees *(pages 124-125)*. This procedure is remarkable for several reasons. It requires some of the most meticulous maneuvers in all of surgery; yet it is highly successful, improving hearing permanently in about 80 per cent of cases. And because it

Replacing the body's smallest bone

Every year, surgery saves thousands from the deafness caused by bony deposits that immobilize the tiny middle-ear bone called, after its shape, the stirrup, or stapes. In a stapedectomy, the operation shown here, the stirrup is replaced with a piston made of plastic too slippery to adhere to bone.

Removal of the natural stirrup, a bone no bigger than a grain of rice, is a miracle of surgical miniaturization. Working under a microscope, the surgeon cuts away most of the stirrup, then makes a hole in its minute footplate, at the entrance to the inner ear; hearing could be destroyed if a slip of an instrument damaged the cochlea, which transmits sound signals to the brain. Finally, the plastic replacement *(opposite, right)* is fitted into place.

Immediately after surgery, the patient can hear again, and hearing generally keeps improving for about a month. One man realized the degree of his recovery a week later, on hearing the roar of a broken air conditioner grinding itself to bits. "Never," he exclaimed, "had I heard such a great sound!"

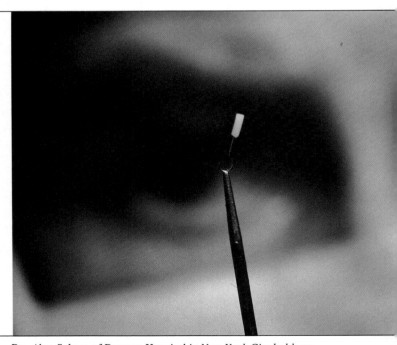

Dr. Alan Scheer of Doctors Hospital in New York City holds an artificial stapes in tweezers just before implanting it in a patient's middle ear. The cylinder, made of the waxy plastic that is used to coat nonstick frying pans, will take the place of the natural bone; the wire hook will hold the cylinder against the anvil, or incus, one of the vibrating bones of the middle ear.

is usually performed under local anesthesia, its results are startlingly immediate.

To enter the middle ear, the surgeon makes a curved incision close to the rim of the eardrum and folds half of the eardrum forward on itself like an omelette. Working under the microscope, with delicate instruments, he breaks off the thin legs of the stirrup where they join the footplate and removes the entire curved piece of bone. Then, using a tiny drill and the tip of a fine curved hook, he pries loose bits of the footplate and removes them with forceps.

When the oval window has been exposed, he is ready to create a new link between the anvil and the inner ear. For this connection he may choose one of several devices; one commonly used is a piece of metal or plastic that looks like a small piston with a hooked wire on top. Very carefully, the surgeon eases the flat base of the piston through the hole chipped in the footplate so that the piston rests in the oval window; at the same time, the wire is hooked over the knobby end of the anvil. Immediately, sound waves can pass through the oval window, and the patient—still on the operating table—suddenly is able to hear again. The noise of the moment may be mundane—the murmuring of nurses, the clink of instruments, the background music of the operating room—but for a patient who is deaf one minute and able to hear the next, they can be the sweetest sounds of a lifetime.

The breakthrough is equally exhilarating for the surgeon, who knows at once that his efforts have been successful. "It's really quite dramatic," Dr. Jerome Goldstein of Albany Medical College said recently. "Many patients you had to shout at when you started to operate can hear a whisper by the time you finish."

Yet for all its drama, the stapedectomy has become almost routine. In little more than a quarter of a century, a major cause of hearing loss has been conquered with bits of plastic and wire—and the Superman vision bestowed by the microscope. What appears an astounding feat to the observer is, to the modern microsurgeon, just the beginning of another workday. ✳

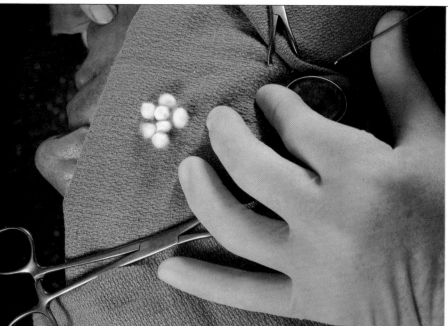

Dr. Scheer inserts the artificial stapes—the white speck visible at top right—into the ear through a speculum, a funnel-shaped instrument that dilates the canal of the outer ear and keeps it open throughout the operation. The tiny cotton swabs are used from time to time to clear the outer-ear canal of blood seeping into it from the middle ear.

ANVIL BONE GROWTH STIRRUP INNER EAR MIDDLE EAR FOOTPLATE

PLASTIC STIRRUP

When the stirrup bone is immobilized by growths, sound cannot reach the inner ear. To restore hearing, all of the stirrup except the footplate is removed. A hole is cut in the footplate, and a plastic piston is set through it to connect anvil to inner ear.

PHOTOGRAPHS BY ALEXANDER TSIARAS

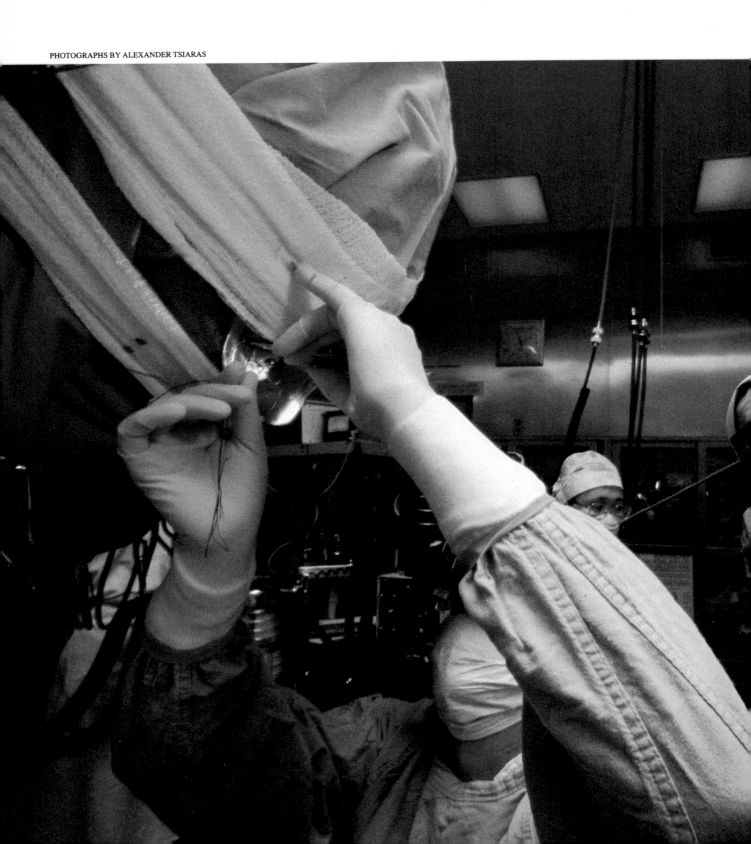

From the operating room, the gift of sight

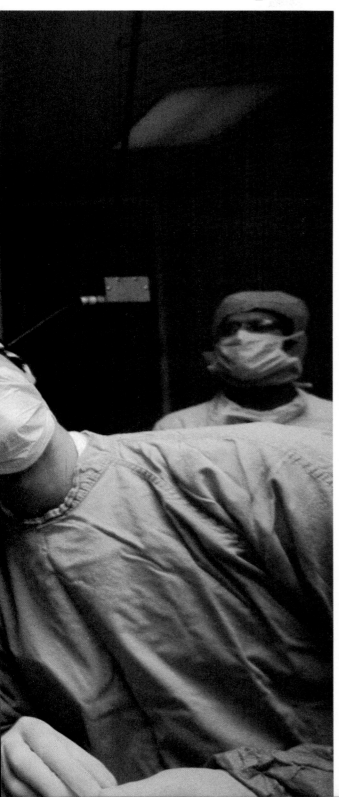

For most of medical history, eye surgery was limited to a single brutal operation practiced as much as 3,000 years ago in India: The physician used a needle to push a cataract-clouded lens out of place and back into the eyeball. In the 18th Century, surgeons learned to cut the lens completely out of the eye so that it could not float back into the pathway of light. But surgical progress stopped there. Not even in the 19th Century, when the structure of the eye was at last fully understood, were there significant advances in tools, techniques or the variety of operations.

Then, beginning in the 1950s, a medical revolution occurred. Over the next quarter century, in an explosion of new discoveries and methods, surgeons explored and corrected the defects of the inner eye, using instruments never before imagined—glass cables that light up the eye's interior, scalpels with blades almost invisible without a microscope, tiny probes that join torn parts with searing heat or freezing cold. Even the operating tables are revolutionary: In the dramatic picture at left, for example, a motor-driven table has turned a patient heels over head, so that gravity can add its force to the treatment of a torn retina.

Today the surgical revolution has made every part of the eye accessible to the surgeon, from the outer crystalline cornea to the light-sensitive retina at the back of the eyeball. Surgeons now can treat injury or disease that threatens vision, and in some cases can literally enable the blind to see.

At the Massachusetts Eye and Ear Infirmary, Dr. H. MacKenzie Freeman reattaches the torn retina of a patient who is strapped head down on a tilted table, only his spotlighted eye and nose uncovered. Dr. Freeman, kneeling on the floor with a retractor in his left hand, pulls with his right hand on threads sewn to the eye muscles, turning the eye while gravity coaxes the retina into normal position (pages 128-129).

A retina reattached by fire and ice

A tiny tear in a cellular layer of the retina—perhaps the size of a pencil point—is fairly common and easily remedied, but if fluid leaks in behind these cells, the layer may flop loose. This is a catastrophe; the torn retina folds over the intact part, threatening total blindness.

The operation shown here reattaches a torn retina by the steps summarized in the drawings opposite. The surgeon begins by replacing the thick vitreous fluid with a thin salt solution, using the technique depicted on pages 134-135. Then, with a heat probe, he sears a string of dotlike scars at the back of the eye as points of attachment for the retina. The most spectacular part of the procedure comes next: He rotates the patient until, by the force of gravity, the retina unfolds back into position. Finally, he ''sews'' the retina firmly in place—not with thread, but by freezing it with a very cold metal probe.

Held fast by straps and pads, an anesthetized patient lies on a motor-driven operating table that can turn or rotate his body to any position.

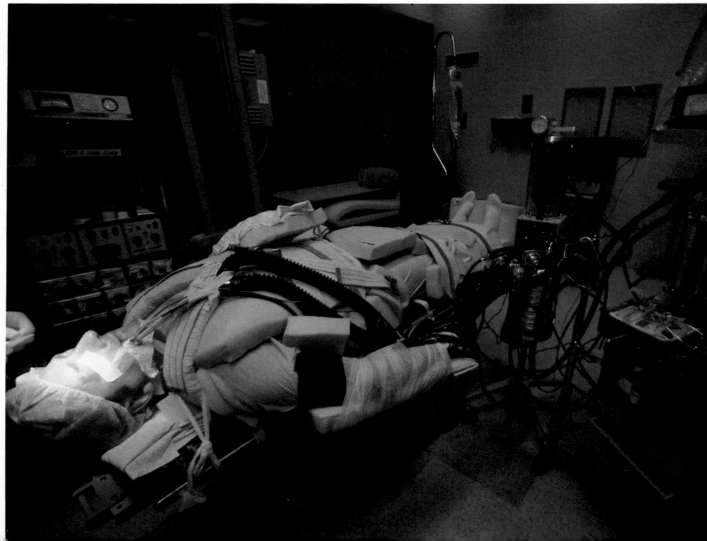

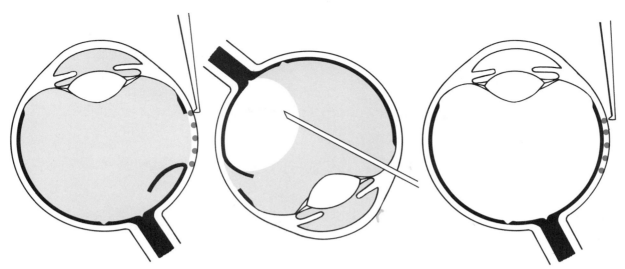

Four skillful hands—belonging to the surgeon and two assistants—perform an intricate ballet. At right, an assistant pulls sutures to turn the patient's eyeball; at left, the surgeon uses a heat probe to burn spots that will help hold the retina.

THREE STEPS TO PUT A RETINA IN PLACE

At far left, above, a torn retina lies folded back as the hot tip of a probe burns attachment points (red dots) in the normal retina position. The patient is turned (center), the retina unfolds, and a needle injects air to flatten the flap. Then a cold probe (right)—at −120° F.—bonds the retina (blue dots).

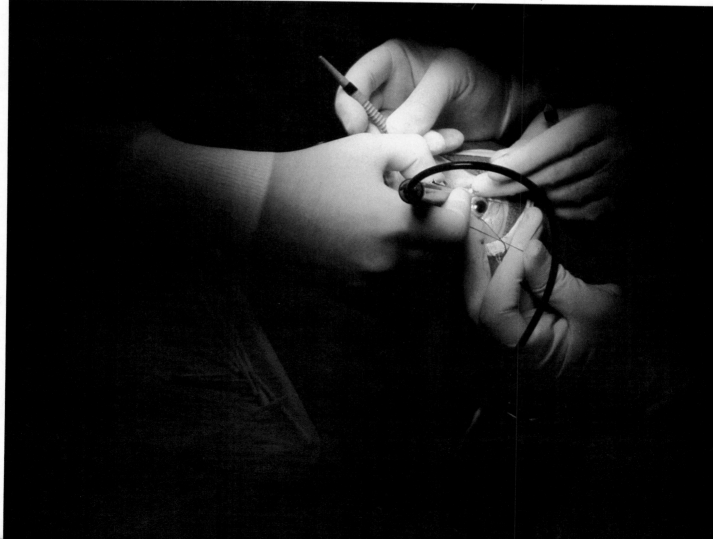

A man-made lens for cataract patients

"It was just like God came over on my side," exulted playwright Leonard Spigelgass. "I was virtually blind, but 12 hours after the 20-minute operation I could see perfectly well." During those 20 minutes Spigelgass, like the patients whose operations are recorded in the pictures at right, had received a complete cure for cataracts, the opacities in the lenses of the eyes that blur or block vision. First, the cataract-clouded lenses were removed; then plastic replacements were put in their place.

Removal of a natural lens leaves the eye unable to focus correctly. Although very thick eyeglasses can correct a lens-less eye, they distort objects and reduce side vision. Contact lenses for cataract patients preserve side vision, but are extremely difficult to insert and remove, especially for elderly people. Plastic implants have neither sort of drawback, and since their introduction in the early 1950s, they have helped revolutionize cataract surgery: By the 1980s, half the 400,000 cataract removals performed annually in the United States were followed by lens implantations.

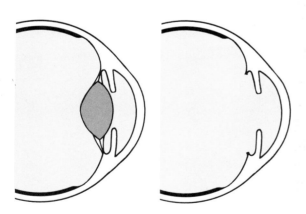

REMOVING THE LENS TO RESTORE VISION
Before surgery (left, above) a cataract-clouded lens (gray) blocks light that passes through the curving cornea toward the interior of the eye; at right, the passageway has been cleared by the removal of the lens. An artificial lens can be implanted either directly in front of the iris or, in the position of the natural lens, behind it.

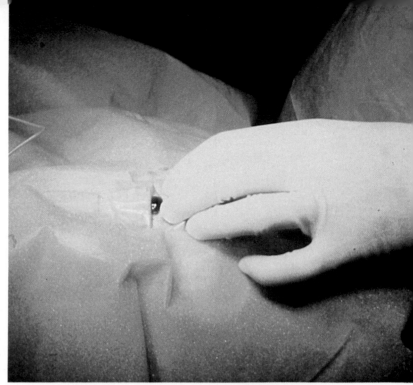

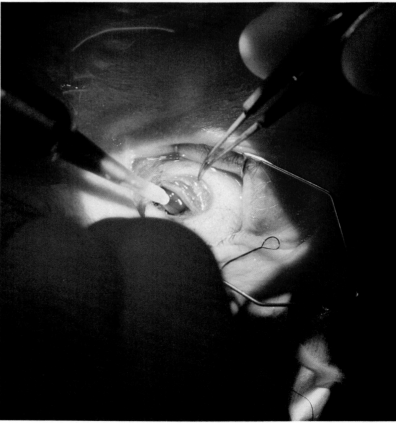

Starting a lens-removal operation (top), a surgeon massages the eyelids to release fluid pressure within the eye. To remove the lens (bottom), he wires the eyelid open, pulls the cornea back with tweezers, then sets the tip of a cold probe against the surface of the lens. The probe and the lens instantly freeze together, and he plucks the lens from the ring of ligaments holding it.

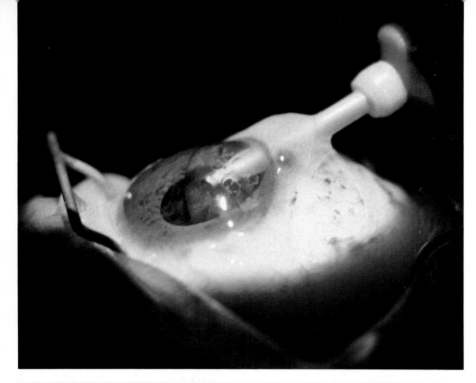

In an alternative removal procedure, a multipurpose tool is inserted into the lens. It emits ultrasonic vibrations to shatter cataracts, then sucks out the disintegrated contents of the lens and injects fluid to maintain pressure in the eyeball. A fairly new technique, emulsification requires only one small incision to gain access to the lens.

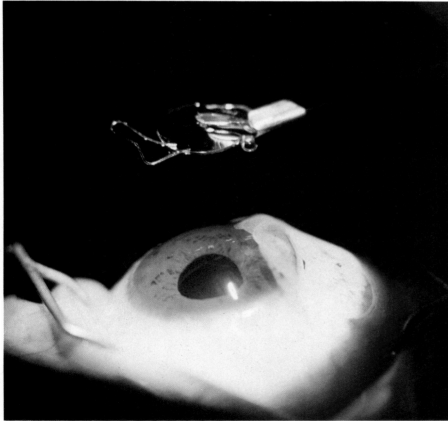

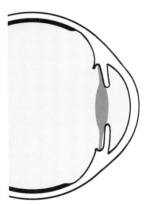

An artificial lens, ready to be implanted, is poised above an eye made lensless by the first stage of cataract surgery. When the substitute is slid into position (drawing, above), the plastic clips attached to it help hold the lens in almost exactly the same location as a natural one.

Building a lens into a cornea

Cornea transplants are not particularly new; surgeons have been using them for decades to replace corneas that are misshapen, scarred or infected. They are new, however, as part of cataract surgery. In the United States, the first operation of the kind shown on these pages was tried in 1977; by 1982, fewer than 150 had been done. Yet the procedure is basically simple, and of great promise.

After removing the lens from the eye of a cataract patient *(preceding pages),* the surgeon takes a slice from a donated cornea, cuts it to a lens shape, then sandwiches it between layers of the patient's own cornea. The corneal section adds its corrective power to that of the patient's cornea, much as an implanted plastic lens would—but with major differences. The operation affects only the tough outer surface of the eye; and because it uses human tissues rather than a foreign body, there is little danger of subsequent irritation.

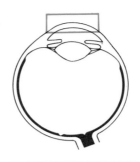

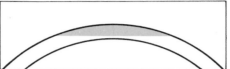

Only the outermost part of a donated cornea, shown in the box at top, is used for a corneal lens. In the enlargement at bottom, the blue shows the part of the cornea that will be taken as raw material for the lens.

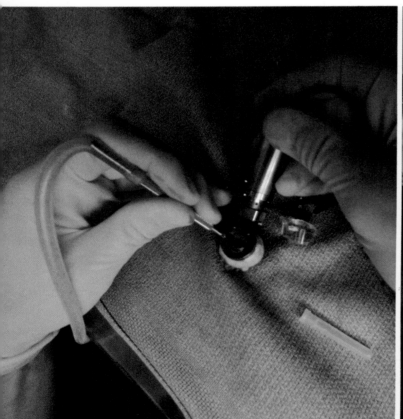

From a cornea willed to an eye bank, a surgeon cuts a slice less than 1/25 inch thick, using a microkeratome—essentially a high-speed oscillating razor. The tool in his left hand does two jobs: It secures the cornea and guides the blade.

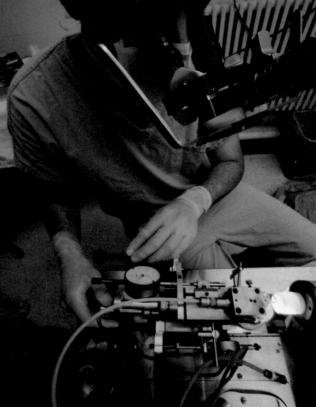

Looking through a microscope, the surgeon uses a miniature lathe to form the cornea—now frozen for rigidity and attached to the bright plastic cylinder at lower right—to a computer-calculated lens shape. Shaping the lens takes less than 45 seconds.

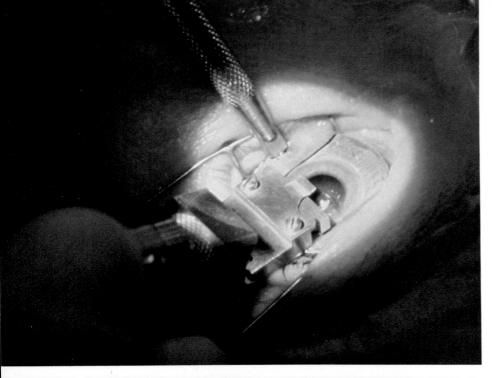

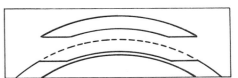

The surgeon now slices off a layer of his patient's cornea (photograph at left and drawing above), using much the same technique as that used on the donated eye (bottom left, opposite).

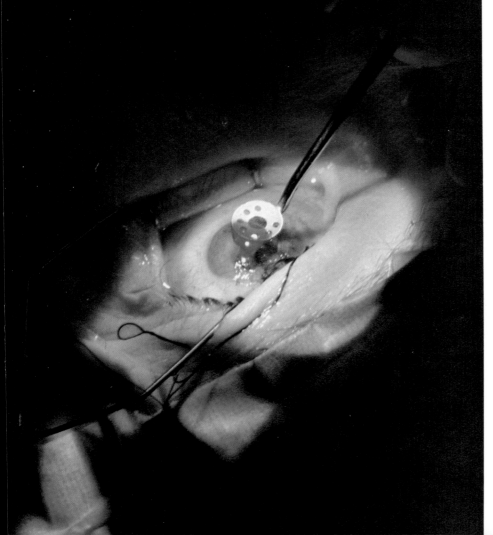

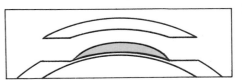

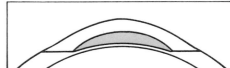

After loosely stitching the patient's cornea section back in place, the surgeon slides the lens-shaped transplant (given a temporary blue tint for visibility) from a tiny spatula to its prepared location; then he will tighten the sutures. The drawings show the parts before (top) and after (bottom) final assembly; the donated cornea is in blue.

Clearing out a clouded fluid

Normally transparent, the thick vitreous fluid that fills most
of the eye can be clouded by hemorrhaging blood or by a
latticework of opaque fibers. No drug will clear it—and as
the eye's interior darkens, vision gradually fails. However,
in a triumph of modern surgery, a way has been found to
replace the vitreous fluid with a liquid clear as glass. The
operation, called a vitrectomy, may be needed to remedy a
defect in the fluid or as part of surgery to reattach a torn retina
(pages 128-129). It may last as long as seven hours.

Two recently developed instruments make this surgery
possible. One is the fiber-optic light pipe—a cable of glass
fibers, each as fine as a human hair, that brings light to the
interior of the eye. The other device is called a VISC, for
Vitreous Infusion Suction Cutter. In a shaft only .066 inch
thick, the VISC does three jobs simultaneously: It cuts and
shreds the vitreous fluid with a rotary blade, sucks the shred-
ded fragments out of the eye, and fills the eyeball with a
transparent salt solution. Later, during the months after a
vitrectomy, the body itself replaces that solution with a clear
solution of its own, secreted at the front of the eye.

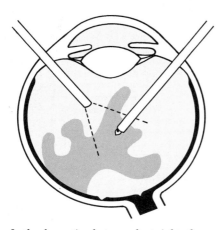

*In the dramatic photograph at right, the
surgeon's left hand holds a fiber-optic pipe
illuminating the eye's interior; in his
right, a VISC replaces the vitreous fluid. The
VISC shaft consists of two concentric
tubes: The inner one cuts and draws out
diseased vitreous fluid (purplish), and the
outer one injects a salt solution.*

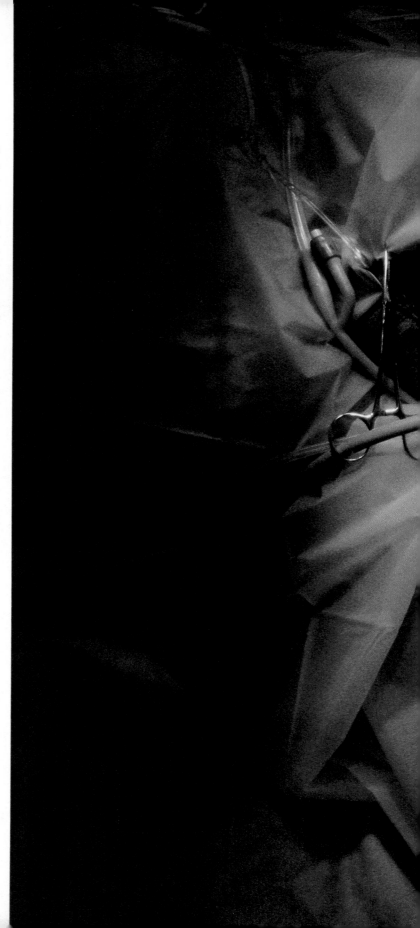

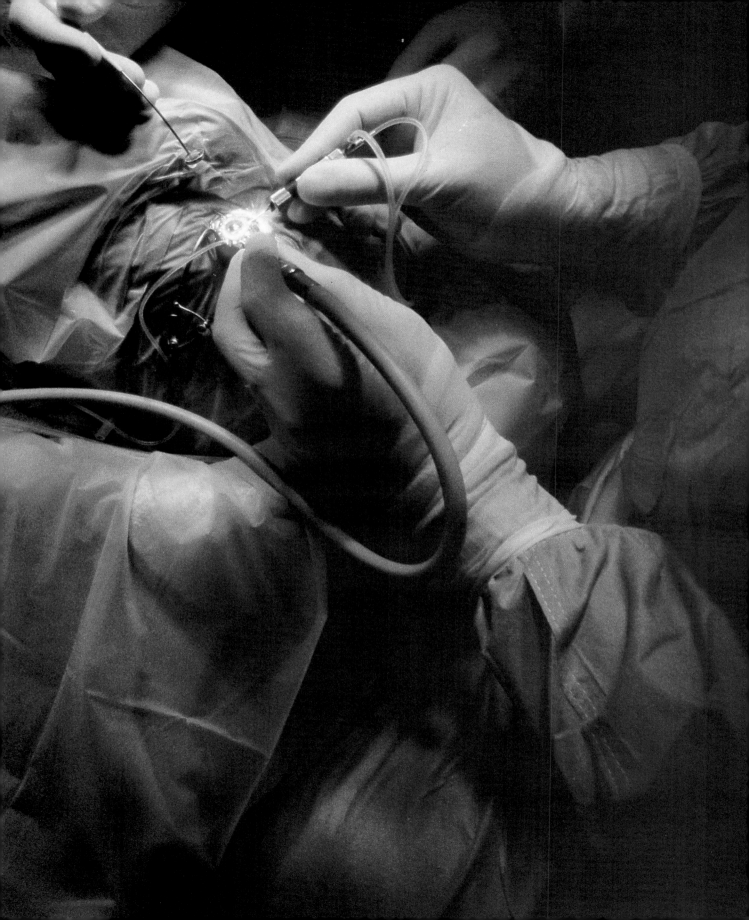

CHAPTER 6

New ways to aid the deaf and blind

Making the most of remaining sight
A sniper's weapon to see in the dark
Inaudible echoes to guide the blind
From talking books to robots that read out loud
Aids for the deaf
Wiring the inner ear for sound

In the past the loss of sight or hearing had to be borne, the handicap seen as a frustrating burden or somehow accepted as a spiritual benefit. Surgery was dangerous and uncertain, eyeglasses and such primitive hearing aids as ear trumpets of limited help.

The English poet John Milton, blinded at the height of his career, had to dictate his later masterpieces to secretaries. He found inner solace. "Why should I not bear gently the deprivation of sight," he wrote in 1656, "when I may hope that it is not so much lost as revoked and retracted inwards, for the sharpening rather than the blunting of my mental image." The composer Ludwig van Beethoven, who wrote many of his greatest works in deafness, was reluctant even to acknowledge his disability. "Alas," he wrote to his brothers in 1802, "how could I declare the weakness of a sense which in me ought to be more acute—a sense which formerly I possessed in the highest perfection."

Were they alive today, neither Beethoven nor Milton would have to view his affliction as inevitable. Handicaps as severe as theirs are being overcome with ingenious devices, mainly the outgrowth of revolutionary discoveries in electronics that followed World War II. If written now, Milton's sonnets and Beethoven's sonatas might pay tribute to such unlikely subjects as microchips, the miniature electronic components that make many of these advances possible.

The idea of using electricity to restore sight and hearing is older than the electronic age itself. In 1751, some 200 years before the transistor was invented, William Watson reported on Benjamin Franklin's lightning experiments to fellow scientists of Britain's Royal Society. In the course of his report he commented on the use of electricity to treat deafness and blindness: "It was imagined that deafness had been relieved by electrising the patient," Watson noted, "and by making him undergo the electrical commotion"—that is, by subjecting him to shocks of static electricity. Just who had devised this treatment, Watson did not say; but evidently he considered the procedure dubious.

In 1800, the Italian scientist Alessandro Volta conducted a daring electrical experiment on his own, normal ears. He set out to see if the sensation of hearing could be produced artificially with electricity. Using the battery he had invented not long before, Volta placed a metal rod in each of his ears, connected them to the terminals with wire and turned on the current. He described the painful result as "a jolt in the head." After the initial shock had worn off, he reported, he heard a bubbling, gurgling sound that reminded him of the "boiling of thick soup." Not surprisingly, Volta's research method failed to inspire imitators, and the auditory aftereffects have never been explained.

The transition from Volta's idea to modern aids was made possible by a range of inventions, largely dependent on electronics but combining advances in such varied fields as optics, computer science, artificial intelligence and surgery. Some of the new devices bolster weakened senses, as spectacles and hearing aids long have done. Others let a working sense substitute for the disabled one—hearing or touch fill-

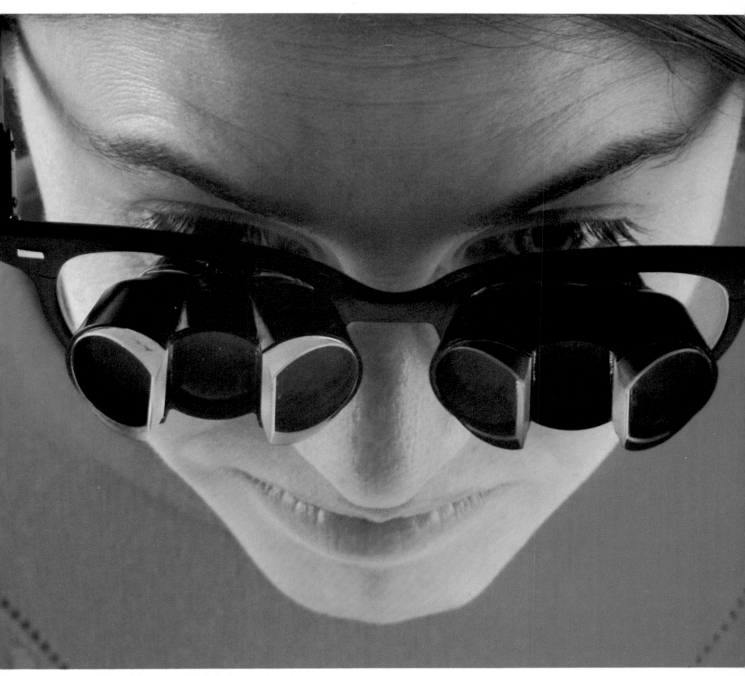

Among new aids to vision are optical devices such as these multilens spectacles, designed for people who have lost sharp central vision. Their three-times magnification enables peripheral vision, much less sharp than central vision, to make out street signs and faces that otherwise would be a blur. Three angled lenses for each eye cover an acceptably broad view.

This leather-encased ear trumpet was made for Ludwig van Beethoven, whose greatest works—the Eroica score is beneath the trumpet—were created after he began to lose his hearing. The bell-like apparatus, which gathered and intensified sounds, helped for a time, but eventually a bone of each middle ear became immobilized, producing total deafness.

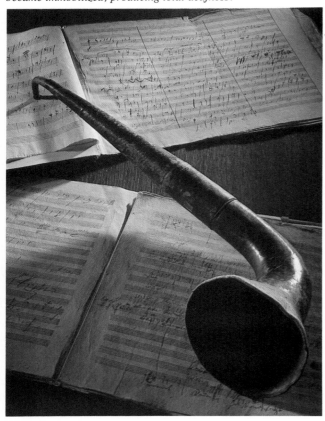

ing in for sight, for example—thus bypassing the handicap. A few feed information directly to brain connections; such devices are, in a very real sense, electronic eyes and ears.

None of this work has produced a true substitute for lost sight or hearing. Nevertheless, today's aids enable many people to hold jobs they otherwise could not, and to achieve fulfillment in life that otherwise would be impossible:

• A blind New Zealander, Wayne Barker, runs a pig farm with the aid of an electronic device that bounces sound off objects and obstacles in his path, enabling him to locate animals, gateways and feeding troughs.

• A deaf lawyer, Michael A. Chatoff, argues a case before the United States Supreme Court with the help of a computer, which translates the court reporter's shorthand into words on a monitor at the lawyer's table.

• In some libraries, blind people listen to books read out loud by a machine.

• A blind factory worker assembles tiny computer parts with the assistance of a miniature television camera that tells him what components it sees on the workbench by tapping out coded messages on his abdomen.

Making the most of remaining sight

Blindness is less common than deafness, but most of the newly devised aids are intended to replace lost vision. They are incredibly diverse. Those that aim to improve existing vision work on simple principles—enlarging or brightening an image until it becomes perceptible. Aids that substitute for vision generally depend on elaborate technology.

Although most people who are called blind can tell light from dark, the images they see are blurred so that the bright parts blend into the dark ones and distinctions among the parts are lost. An *E* on a printed page looks like an *F,* and the features of a face become too hazy to recognize. If the image is enlarged, however, the bright parts and dark parts become big enough to stand out separately: An *E* is seen to have three distinct crossbars. Thus, simple enlargement may be enough to enable a legally blind person to read books, recognize friends and make out signs or obstacles on the street.

Ordinary hand-held magnifiers have long been used in this way, of course, and binoculars or telescopic lenses—which may even be attached to regular spectacle frames—serve the same purpose. But telescopic lenses have a serious limitation: As magnification increases, the field of vision narrows. In 1981, however, Dr. William Feinbloom of the Pennsylvania College of Optometry in Philadelphia devised spectacles with three telescopic lenses for each eye, one pointing forward, two angled to the sides, their images fused into a single, panoramic view that broadens the field of vision as much as six times *(page 137).* One wearer, a college student, improved his vision from 9 per cent of normal to 95 per cent. He can now read a blackboard, see street signs, enjoy baseball games and concert performances and recognize the smiles on his friends' faces. "I'm seeing a lot of things I didn't even know were there."

To aid reading and writing, a number of specialized enlarging devices—some portable but none small enough to be wearable—have been built from electronic components *(pages 148-149)*. They employ closed-circuit television systems or, in one case, an optical scanner somewhat similar to those that read price codes in supermarkets. All enlarge print or handwriting and display the large type on a screen or monitor, permitting people with partial sight to read print made as much as 64 times larger than the original size.

A sniper's weapon to see in the dark

An enlarged image may not suffice for victims of retinitis pigmentosa, the disease that causes total blindness but begins with a gradual loss in sensitivity to dim light. Such people soon become night-blind, unable to find their way in faint illumination—outdoors at night, for example, or even in a candlelit restaurant. To their aid in overcoming this initial handicap has come a civilian version of military equipment such as the Snooperscope and Sniperscope, developed during World War II to enable soldiers to see and shoot accurately in the dark, and since then widely used by astronomers to study faint stars.

The night-vision aid is an image-intensifier. It amplifies light electronically to make a dim view bright. Incoming light, focused by a lens, strikes a photo cathode, a surface that converts light into electricity. Wherever a light ray strikes, the cathode emits one particle of electricity—an electron. Immediately behind the cathode is a glass disk perforated by about a million tiny holes. Electrons from the cathode enter these holes and in passing through bounce against the sides of the holes, at each bounce knocking an additional electron loose from the glass. As a result a single electron triggers a cascade of secondary electrons in the hole, and each electron emitted by the cathode is multiplied into many electrons as it passes through the disk. In this way, the weak energy of dim light is amplified into a relatively powerful current of electrical energy.

The multiplied streams of electrons emerging from the million holes in the disk then strike a phosphor-coated screen, similar to those used in television sets. The phosphor emits light when struck by electrons, converting the electronic signal back into a light image. This final image, as much as 800 times brighter than the original, is then viewed through an eyepiece, enabling many night-blind people to function independently in poor light so long as they retain some of their vision. "I can go fishing again at dusk or dawn," said one man. "I can walk through a restaurant without bumping into chairs and people, and when I get to my table, I can read the menu for myself."

If eyes have lost nearly all their power, brightening or enlarging an image serves no purpose. The eyes then must be bypassed and information about the surrounding world transmitted to the brain in some other way. Touch and hearing are the principal means by which blind individuals navigate, avoid hazards, recognize objects and even, with outside help, assimilate information from books.

Using touch for sight

Touch is the basic substitute for sight. The blind individual feels his way, not only with his feet and hands but with their extension, the cane. Touch began to be used for reading in France as early as 1784, when Valentin Haüy printed raised letters on paper, a scheme later converted into a code of six raised dots and in 1824 given essentially its present form (and its name) by Louis Braille, a blind teacher and musician. Interpreting the braille code, one letter at a time, is rewarding but tedious. And encoding material into braille is time- and paper-consuming: Since the embossed patterns must be large enough for identification by fingertips, braille manuscripts may need 10 times as much paper as the printed original.

In 1976 French scientists Andrée and Oleg Tretiakoff eliminated the paper, replacing it with cassette recording tape that could send signals to a special braille display board. Since computer programs are stored on magnetic tape, it seemed logical to the Tretiakoffs that signals representing braille letters could also be recorded on tape.

Several manufacturers now make tape recorder-players that serve as ordinary sound machines but also accept and produce signals in braille. In addition to the usual loudspeaker, these paperless braille readers have a reading board of 24 or more groups of retractable metal pins, each group containing six pins. The pins pop up and down in the standard braille patterns as the tape plays: A group with a pin projecting in the upper left means *a* and two upper-left pins mean *b*, while all six pins raised stand for the word "for." The blind user runs fingers across the board from left to right, reading a couple of dozen letters at a time.

These paperless readers record braille onto tape. And they permit a blind person to interact with the machine, requesting specific information and definitions instead of simply reading a prerecorded tape. They have computerized memories and keyboards for locating and calling up specific information. In one type a prerecorded dictionary tape can be inserted, enabling the user to key in a word he does not understand and within 30 seconds read the definition of that word on the braille display board.

The entire task of encoding written material into braille, which severely limits the literature available to blind people, is bypassed by another machine, the brain child of electrical engineer John Linvill of Stanford University, whose daughter was born blind but with her parents' help grew up to earn her Ph.D. in psychology. In it, a television camera scans the page electronically and, unlike the paperless braille machines, presents the words one letter at a time. But instead of a pattern of braille dots, the actual shape of a letter or number is traced on the index finger by a grid of 144 movable pins. After a year of practice, a user can read 60 words per minute; by comparison, a sighted high-school student reads 250 to 450 words per minute.

This time-consuming process may not be suitable for reading works of literature, but it can be invaluable for reading documents not usually available in braille: bank statements, bills and typed letters. And because the device reproduces the actual shape of each figure it sees, it can be used to read foreign scripts and mathematical formulas.

An aid that in some ways is more versatile operates in a similar fashion but conveys information to the skin of the abdomen and back rather than to the fingertip. Developed at San Francisco's Smith-Kettlewell Institute of Visual Sciences by Dr. Carter C. Collins and his associates, it has a miniature television camera mounted on an eyeglass frame. A wire carries the TV signals to a skin-tight vest worn under a shirt. Embedded in the vest are 1,024 tiny silver electrodes arranged in a grid of 32 rows of 32 each. If the camera is pointed toward a horizontal bar, then electrodes tracing the outline of a horizontal bar will be turned on. The electrodes vibrate against the skin so that the user feels the outline, as if it was being dotted on the skin by the tip of a ballpoint pen.

Because the device activates so many pins, it can trace objects of more varied shapes than printed letters. And because it is portable, it can be used almost like eyes to visualize anything in the surroundings. Using this substitute vision, one man, blind from the age of three months, has been able to make out his own hand for the first time, to recognize faces and to follow the movement of other people.

Using sound for sight

Although the sense of touch helps some blind people read and move about, the sense of hearing can be made even more useful as a substitute for vision. If books and signs can be made to speak, and objects to announce their presence with sounds, then blind individuals can orient and educate themselves without having to rely on the relatively crude perceptions of touch. A number of new devices supplement the cane by using sound to detect and warn of obstacles in a blind person's path. Moreover, talking signs announce the locations of doorways, elevators and restrooms at the press of a button; and computers now read books to blind listeners in synthetic but clearly understandable speech.

Sounds help everyone, blind or sighted, in moving about; some objects make noise and others betray their location by the echoes they create. The blind person's cane, in fact, is used not simply to extend the sense of touch but also to generate echoes with sharp taps against a floor or pavement. The echoes of footsteps can serve the same purpose. By listening to the echoes, a blind individual can learn to tell when he is coming close to a wall and even when he is emerging from a confined space into an open area—as when he reaches the end of a block lined with buildings and arrives at an intersection.

The audible echoes made in these ways can detect only large objects, such as walls or perhaps a partly closed door; a blind individual cannot tell from ordinary echoes that a chair blocks the path. The reason is the relatively long wave length of audible sounds; a wave is sharply reflected only from objects that are bigger than its own wave length.

This phenomenon was illustrated by writer Isaac Asimov, with the example of a driver searching for a curbside parking place by listening to the echoes of engine noise. Asimov explained, "When driving along a line of irregularly parked cars, we can, if we listen, easily tell the difference in the engine sound of our own car as we pass parked cars and the engine sound as we pass empty parking places. In the former case the engine sound has its echo added, and there would be no difficulty in locating, through the contrast, an unoccupied parking place with our eyes closed. Unfortunately, we could not tell whether that unoccupied parking place had a fireplug or not. A car is large enough to reflect the wave lengths of some of our engine noises but a fireplug is not. To detect objects smaller than a car would require sound waves of shorter wave length."

Sound waves of short wave length do indeed make echoes that are useful in locating objects. Some animals, such as bats and dolphins, employ them instead of vision to find their way and to hunt food. Bats are not totally blind. However, they rely almost entirely on these so-called ultrasonics—sounds of such short wave lengths (and consequently high frequencies) that they are inaudible to humans. As a bat flies, it emits a series of high-pitched squeaks, which bounce off even tiny insects to be picked up by the bat's oversized ears. The bat, by judging the time taken for the echo to return, along with the sound's relative loudness and strength in each ear, can tell not only where the object is but also what it is.

Inaudible echoes to guide the blind

Ultrasonic echolocation was invented by human engineers about the same time scientists discovered that the same scheme had evolved naturally in bats and other animals. The

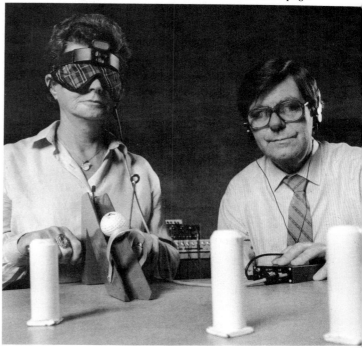

Leslie Kay instructs his wife, Nora, a teacher of blind children, in using a headband vision aid he developed. Like many similar devices, it bounces sound waves off objects and picks up echoes that help the wearer judge the size and distance of objects. Monitoring her skill, Nora Kay listens in on the signals that enable her, while blindfolded, to aim a ball to knock down pegs.

man-made system—sonar—was first developed just before World War II to locate submarines. Soon after the War, a number of engineers in many parts of the world began to develop sonar devices to guide blind people.

One aid that comes close to duplicating the bat's sound-location system, the Sonicguide, is the invention of British-born electrical engineer Leslie Kay, who had worked on sonar instruments to help Royal Navy divers and submariners detect objects on the sea bed and inspect damaged ship hulls. Inspiration for the Sonicguide came when Kay read a newspaper article about the opening of a swimming pool for blind children. "I tried to imagine the problem of a blind child when he set out to swim in any particular direction," said Kay not long ago, "and I realized that what I had been doing for the Navy divers could be relevant."

The miniature working parts of the guide that Kay and his associates later perfected in New Zealand are incorporated into a spectacle frame, so that a blind wearer can use the same head movements as a sighted person to scan the surroundings. An ultrasonic transmitter is built into the center of the frame, and reflected pulses of sound are picked up by two receivers, one mounted on each side of the transmitter. Because the ultrasonic pulses are inaudible, the receivers transform them into electrical signals, then process the signals and channel them to earphones—the right-side receiver to the right earphone, left to left.

The user determines the distance of an obstacle by the pitch of the electronically processed signal. Objects at the maximum range of about 20 feet generate high-pitched signals, while closer obstructions are revealed by signals of gradually lower pitch. Direction is determined by the relative loudness of the echo signals over the earphones: Objects located to the right send stronger signals to the right ear. With training and experience, users can even gauge the texture of an obstacle, using that information to differentiate between a smooth-surfaced glass window and a rough-textured concrete wall; smooth surfaces reflect most of the ultrasonic pulse, while rough surfaces break up and dissipate it. Over the earphones, the differences are subtle but distinguishable: The smooth surface's signal is a purer, clearer tone, slightly different in pitch from the signal of a textured surface.

The short wave lengths of the ultrasonic sounds employed in such guidance devices focus sharply enough to detect fairly small objects—a fireplug, a chair or even a step. Shorter wave lengths would provide even sharper focusing for more precise guidance, and one new aid uses light waves from a laser—perhaps 100 million times shorter than ultrasonic waves. But all these devices can convey information only crudely, making buzzes or beeps that are difficult to interpret, and at best give a rough idea of the facts of the situation. Much better would be a voice, communicating information in speech.

From talking books to robots that read out loud

A few talking machines have been developed. Among them are such everyday conveniences as bathroom scales, clocks, calculators and electronic games. The talking calculator, for example, gives a running commentary on calculations, con-firming each number and function as keys are pressed, and announcing the result over a speaker.

Although talking calculators are new, talking books and magazines have been available since the 1930s. They, too, have been made more useful by developments in electronics. Listening to tapes ordinarily takes much longer than reading by sight: Most tapes recite only 150 words per minute, as compared with the 250 to 450 words per minute that sighted people can read visually. Sighted people can also vary the reading pace at will. To give blind individuals this versatility, engineers have devised speech compressors.

Increasing the tape speed is not enough. Changes in speed create changes in pitch that reduce speech to gibberish. Instead, tiny portions of the speech itself must be blocked electronically at predetermined intervals. Most speakers, for example, articulate words at much greater length than is necessary for comprehension. By clipping off bits of that articulation, engineers can speed up the tape and still keep the words intelligible. At full speed, a speech compressor can whiz through a taped book at some 375 words per minute, a pace comparable to that of sighted people.

Although tape compressors and paperless braille readers can increase the speed at which blind people can listen to talking books or read braille, transcriptions cannot keep pace with the flood of printed matter in today's world; for example, 40,000 books are published each year in the United States alone. Less than 5 per cent of this deluge is put into braille or onto tape in a given year. The ultimate reading machine, then, is one that requires neither tape nor touch—a machine capable of reading any printed material in its original form and translating the print directly into spoken English. This was exactly the challenge taken up by Raymond Kurzweil while he was a student in the Artificial Intelligence Laboratory at Massachusetts Institute of Technology. Kurzweil set out to write a computer program that would enable a machine to recognize letters in any size or style of print and then say the words out loud.

Until then, computers had been programed to recognize the signals generated by electronically scanning special type, such as the letters and numbers that banks print on checks so that they can be processed by machine. Kurzweil aimed to break down each letter into a series of geometric patterns that could be recognized no matter what type they were printed in. A capital *A*, for example, consists of an upper triangle—completely enclosed—and two lower extensions, the triangle sides, with an open space at the bottom. In all the type styles ordinarily used, these three elements—the enclosed area, the extensions and the open space—always exist in that relationship; they occur in no other letter.

Most of the other letters have distinctive shapes and thus can be easily identified in a computer program. In some cases, however, two different letters may look much the same, and to enable the computer to tell which is which, Kurzweil had to include a circuit he calls a disambiguator. He recently explained how it distinguishes between a capital, or upper-case, *I* and a small, or lower-case, *l:*

"If there is a space to the left and the right, it is most likely an upper-case *I* (in fact the word "I"). If there is a space to the left and a consonant to the right, it is again probably an upper-case *I* because there do not exist very many words starting with *l* with second-letter consonants. Number context must also be taken into consideration to deal with the possibility of its being the number one."

With the character-recognition problem solved, Kurzweil then programed the computer to group the letters into words and then to find in its memory their correct pronunciation. He and his colleagues broke the English language into 1,000 sound combinations and catalogued some 1,500 exceptions to the normal rules of pronunciation. In use, letter groups are routed first to the dictionary of exceptions. If none of these applies, the letter groups are shunted to the file of standard pronunciations and electronically transformed into sound by tone generators that follow the computer's instructions to synthesize human speech. The machine sounds like the robot it is, but its reading out loud is easily understood.

Aids for the deaf

Machines that help blind people are in some ways easier to devise than those for deaf persons. Only a few aids to speech comprehension have been invented, with limited success.

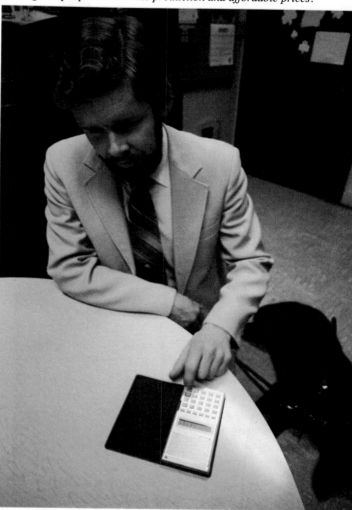

David Loux, a blind representative of the organization that trains Seeing Eye dogs like the Labrador at his side, computes with a talking calculator that he uses in his job. Such calculators, which speak the numbers displayed on their screens, were once costly aids for the blind, but their popularity with sighted people led to mass production and affordable prices.

In 1967, Hubert Upton walked into a conference of the National Institutes of Health wearing what appeared to be an ordinary pair of spectacles. But built into one of the lenses was a tiny mirror that reflected rapid flashes of light into Upton's eye. A wire from the frame ran to a small electronic gadget that bulged from his pocket.

The gadget in Upton's pocket was a speech analyzer, connected to a microphone in his tie clip that picked up the words of nearby persons. The analyzer distinguished characteristics of speech, such as pitch, and the sounds of vowels and fricative consonants such as *f*. The signals turned on tiny lights in his eyeglass frames, making the flashes that were reflected off the mirror. When Upton aligned his glasses correctly, the flashes appeared to be emanating from the speaker's mouth, their pattern providing clues to the letters spoken. In later, more sophisticated models, a yellow light, flashed in the upper portion of his field of vision, told Upton that he was seeing an *e* sound, while a red light meant *s* or *z*, and green stood for *u* or *o*.

After using various versions of the device continuously, Upton became so accustomed to the display that he was barely conscious of any interference with his normal vision. But over the years, according to Dr. Blair F. Simmons of Stanford University, no one other than Upton has been able to master this complex lip-reading aid.

The sense of touch is also being explored as an aid to lip reading. At the University of Texas, Brian Scott developed three flat plastic vibrators, each about the size of a silver dollar, that are worn on a belt around the waist. The middle disk responds only to high-frequency sounds, such as the sound of *s*. The two outer vibrators respond simultaneously to *sh* sounds, while all three disks vibrate simultaneously to indicate vowel sounds such as *o* and *u*.

Wiring the inner ear for sound

The ultimate aid for deaf or blind people would be electronic eyes or ears that served as genuine replacements for the natural sense organs: a television camera connected to the vision center of the brain, a microphone connected to the hearing center. Both have been made, the substitute for hearing thus far proving more successful than the one for sight.

After Alessandro Volta's jolting experiment in 1800, little was done to send sound by electricity directly to the brain, until 1957. In that year, Dr. A. Djourno and his colleagues in France restored some hearing to a deafened man by implanting an electrode near his auditory nerve, connecting it to a receiving coil implanted under the skin, and relaying signals to the coil electromagnetically.

The electronic ear

If all the usual remedies prove futile, a deaf individual may now be able to regain some hearing with an electronic ear, an artificial substitute organ that is connected to the auditory nerve. The system has both implanted and external components. Sound is detected by a microphone set in the ear, and is converted into electrical signals by a pocket-sized processing unit. A wire connects the processor to a transmitting coil mounted near the ear—generally on eyeglass frames. This coil relays the signals electromagnetically to a receiving coil implanted under the skin above and behind the ear, and another wire carries the signals from there to the cochlea, stimulating the auditory nerve.

The sounds conveyed by these electronic components are crude compared to those perceived in normal hearing. The wearer is not able to understand individual spoken words, but can often distinguish differences among music, speech and such environmental sounds as a siren or doorbell.

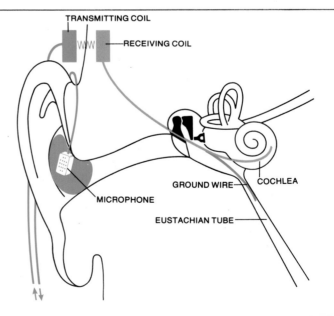

Sound picked up by a microphone goes to a processing unit (not shown), then to the transmitting coil. There, the electrical signals generate electromagnetic waves (blue zigzag), which, unimpeded by skin, induce identical signals in a coil wired to the cochlea.

Variations of this technique *(pages 144-145),* which can restore some hearing even to those who have suffered previously untreatable damage to the inner-ear mechanism, have since been used on several hundred patients by a number of surgeons. However, the operation requires delicate surgery, risking damage to the brain, and it restores hearing only in some cases, and then to a limited degree.

Yet for many people who cannot hear even with the most powerful hearing aids, the implants have provided enough sound, however tinny and fluctuating, to help them use lip reading to interpret conversations. "I can hear others around me talking," said one patient after the device was implanted, "so I don't interrupt their conversations. If I know the topic of the conversation, every once in a while I can get the words. I still have to rely mainly on lip reading."

Hearing that is even less distinct can also be helpful. "When I was out, I worried that I had left the garbage disposal on at home—I have burned out a few disposals because I could not hear them running," said one woman recently. "I always wanted to go back home to make sure that everything

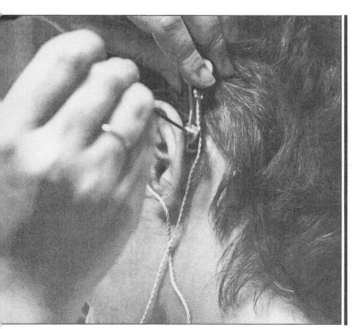

Holding the white disk of a transmitter with a forefinger, an audiologist adjusts its position on its eyeglass support. Alignment of this outer coil over the receiving coil implanted within the skull is crucial to electromagnetic transmission of the signal.

was all right." After the implant surgery, she gained confidence. "When I'm driving by myself, I can hear sirens. I don't know what direction they are coming from, but I can pull to the side of the road. I can even tell when something sounds wrong with my car."

These results have been achieved through the use of a single electrode connected at one point on the auditory nerve. At the University of Utah, Stanford University, the University of California in San Francisco and the University of Washington in Seattle, experimental implants have employed eight separate channels—as many as can, with existing techniques, be wired into the tiny area in which the electrodes must be placed. These multichannel implants make it possible for patients to understand about half the common words used in conversation.

The modest success of the electronic ear cannot yet be matched by an electronic eye, although experimental devices have been implanted in several blind volunteers by Dr. William H. Dobelle of Columbia University. The most promising results were obtained in the case of a young man who had been blinded 10 years earlier by a gunshot wound. A group of 64 electrodes were implanted in the vision center of his brain and wired to a connector outside his skull, behind his right ear. To this connector was plugged a computer that received signals from a television camera. When an impulse was fed to a brain electrode it produced a sensation—the perception of a spot of light—that seemed to the blind man to be in one place; the spot generated by each electrode always appeared in the same position.

Thus the camera view could be processed by the computer to generate an image in the volunteer's brain. He could not distinguish pictures or letters, but he could tell horizontal bars from vertical bars, and he could perceive the dots of a braille pattern visually. In fact, he read braille with the electronic eye five times faster than he could with his fingers.

Crude as electronic substitutes for eyes and ears are now, they work. That fact alone shows how much progress has been made in providing artificial aids for deficient senses. The help that Milton and Beethoven could hardly have dreamed of, let alone hoped for, is clearly ahead. ✳

Machines that see

Futuristic devices that use laser beams, inaudible sound waves, synthetic speech and microcomputers promise to make it easier for blind people to overcome their most formidable handicaps: the difficulties of reading and of getting about in a labyrinthine world of unseen obstacles. Learning to master these devices—many of which communicate what they read or observe by such unfamiliar means as beeps, buzzes and tickles—requires specialized training at such institutions as the Perkins School for the Blind and the Carroll Center for the Blind, shown on the following pages. Here, blind people work with student teachers from nearby Boston College in applying the new tools as supplements to the traditional braille, long cane and guide dog, which are still the basic, indispensable substitutes for vision.

Most of the new mobility devices depend on ultrasonic detection techniques adapted from submarine sonar, in which sound so high-pitched it cannot be heard is bounced off solid objects and reveals their locations by the echoes. An exception is a laser-powered cane, which also locates obstacles by reflection but employs invisible light waves instead of inaudible sound.

The reading aids are of two types. Print enlargers, designed for people who have limited vision, scan text and flash the words—enormously magnified—on a screen. For the totally blind, some devices communicate the text by tapping on the skin, and complex computers versed in English linguistics read out loud absolutely anything they are given.

High cost and complexity limit the use of most of these new aids. Generally they find temporary application in helping the blind adjust to their handicap; some are so expensive they are found only in institutions.

At the Carroll Center for the Blind, near Boston, a student instructor shows how to locate a brief case on the floor with a hand-held sensor that emits inaudible sound. The sound, bounced back by the obstacle, causes the sensor to vibrate.

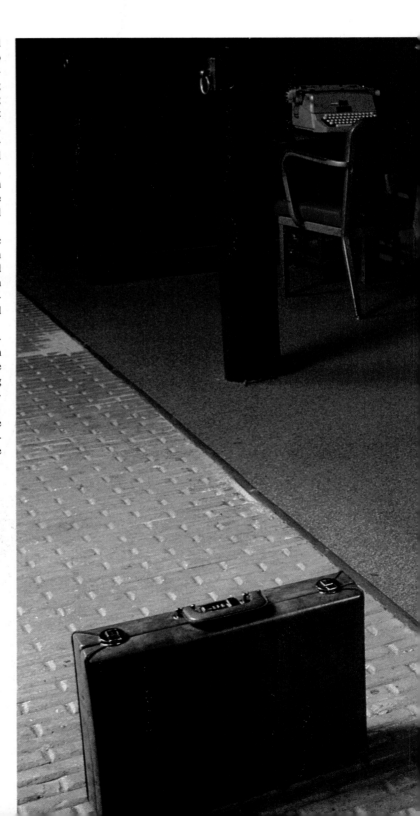

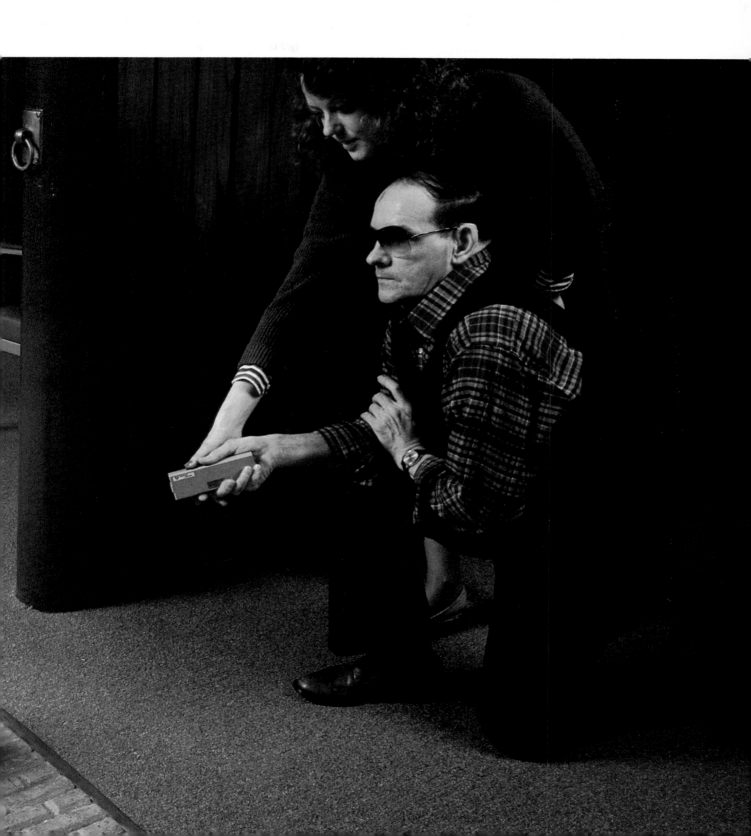

New ways to read the printed word

Aids in reading have long been a high-priority concern of blind people. Now several devices, making use of technology from diverse fields, supplement scarce braille texts and talking books.

The simplest of these new reading aids are enlargers, meant for people who are partially blind. Two devices pictured here scan any kind of print or handwriting, then display the image as much as 64 times larger on a screen.

An electronic alternative for someone who is totally blind is the complex but surprisingly compact talking reader at far right. Outwardly resembling a small office copying machine, it recognizes printed words as clusters of phonetic sounds and then synthesizes the words electronically, reading aloud in English—albeit with something like a Swedish accent. To deal with the myriad irregularities of English pronunciation and spelling, its memory banks are crammed with 1,000 rules and 1,500 exceptions to them. It even has an embossing attachment that automatically converts the printed text into a braille tape for those who are deaf as well as blind.

The hand-held scanner of the Viewscan system being used at right contains some 500 fine glass fibers to relay light from the printed page to an electronic chip, which senses light or dark from one fiber at a time in rapid succession. The chip signals the screen to turn on or off pinpoints of neon light, crudely reproducing the type. The knob at bottom right adjusts magnification.

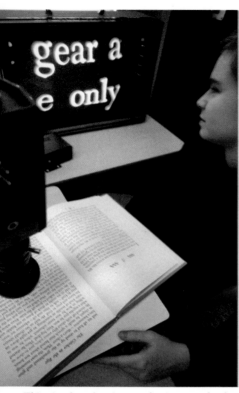

This simple enlarging reader is a standard closed-circuit television system— a camera connected to a television set. The camera is focused for extreme close-ups, and it gives a detailed image, enlarged 32 times, of anything placed in its field of view.

A blind woman adjusts a Kurzweil Reading Machine as it reads aloud the book placed face down over its scanner. The scanner's 512 photocells—each .00008 inch wide—signal light or dark to the computer, which combines pieces of letters to recognize characters, groups letters into words, searches its memory for pronunciation, then synthesizes sounds.

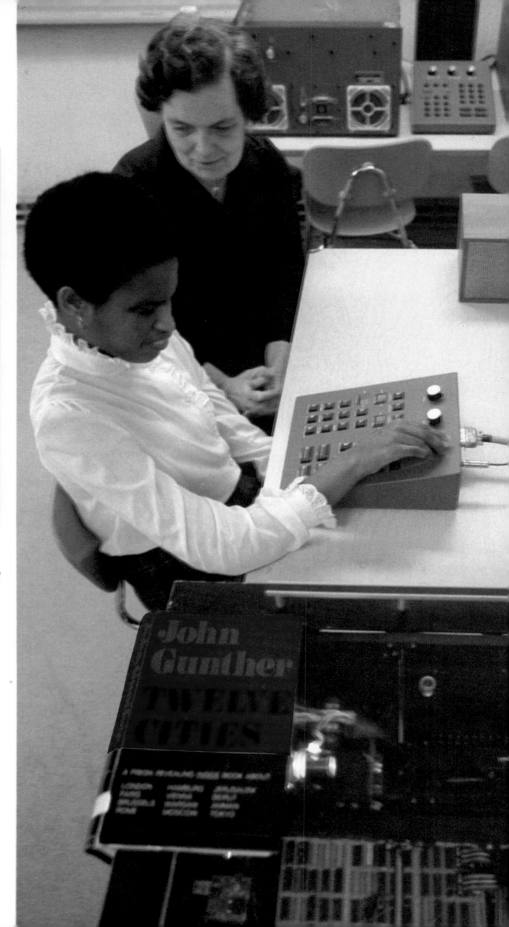

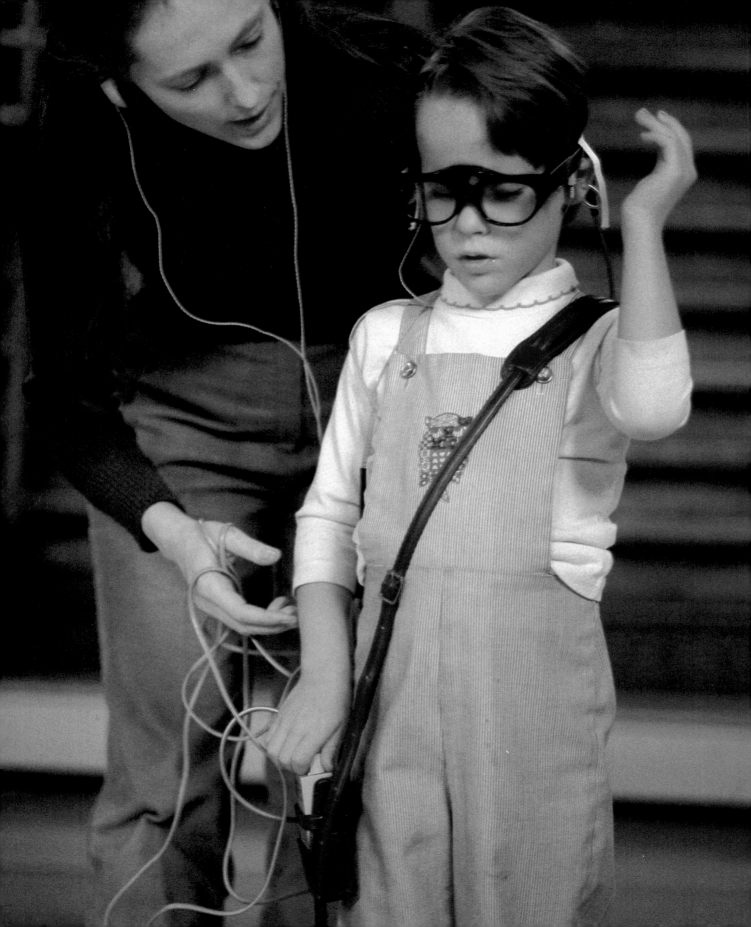

Echoes to walk around by

Blind people have always used the echoes of their cane taps to help them find their way, but a number of new pathfinders locate obstacles more precisely. All are small and easy to carry. The type in these two pictures, relying on the ultrasonic echoes of inaudible sound waves, fits into a spectacle frame *(left);* another, which picks up the reflections of a laser beam, is built into a standard white long cane.

The obstacle finders use various means to tell what they ''see.'' A hand-held ultrasonic sensor *(pages 147 and 152)* vibrates when the emitted sound echoes off an object; the closer the obstacle, the harder the sensor shakes. A sensor worn on a neck strap vibrates against the chest and neck to alert those both blind and deaf, but also beeps, its pitch ascending as the user draws nearer to the object.

The spectacle-frame sensor has two angled receivers that can convey a different signal, converted into audible sound, to each ear, thus indicating the direction of the hazard. The object's distance and even its texture are revealed by changes in the sound's pitch and timbre. The laser device uses all the means of communication—varying tones, beeps and vibrations—to advise of obstacles straight ahead, at ground level and at head height.

A five-year-old girl, blind since birth, raises her hand for her ultrasonic glasses to detect so that she can adjust the device. Her teacher listens through duplicate earphones to signals generated when sounds aimed from the center of the eyeglass frames bounce back to adjacent receivers.

Negotiating an icy sidewalk, a young woman uses her ultrasonic eyeglasses to find a stoplight post. A distinctive beep begins to sound in her earphones when she approaches to within about 15 feet of an obstacle such as the post.

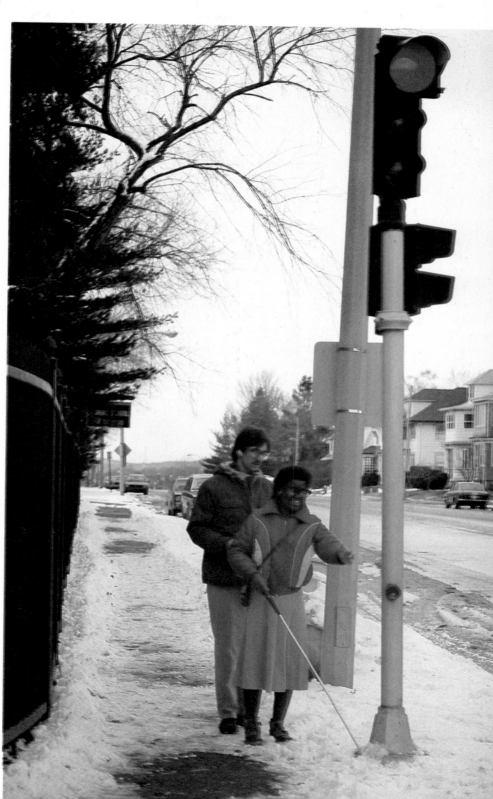

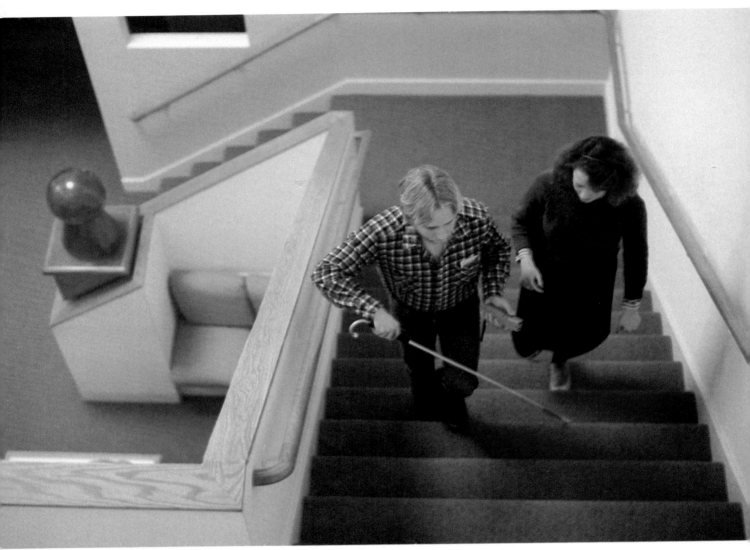

*Practicing a navigating technique known as shorelining—
following a wall by means of an ultrasonic sensor—a blind man
climbs a flight of stairs, helped by a student teacher. This
pathfinding device, called a Mowat Sensor, transmits a constant
level of vibrations to the hand when the user keeps to a straight
line; the signal intensity changes if he deviates.*

*Guided by an ultrasonic Pathsounder
worn around his neck, a man finds his way
around a roomful of obstacles in a
workshop for the blind. The device leaves
one hand free to check for hazards such
as the pole and the workbench.*

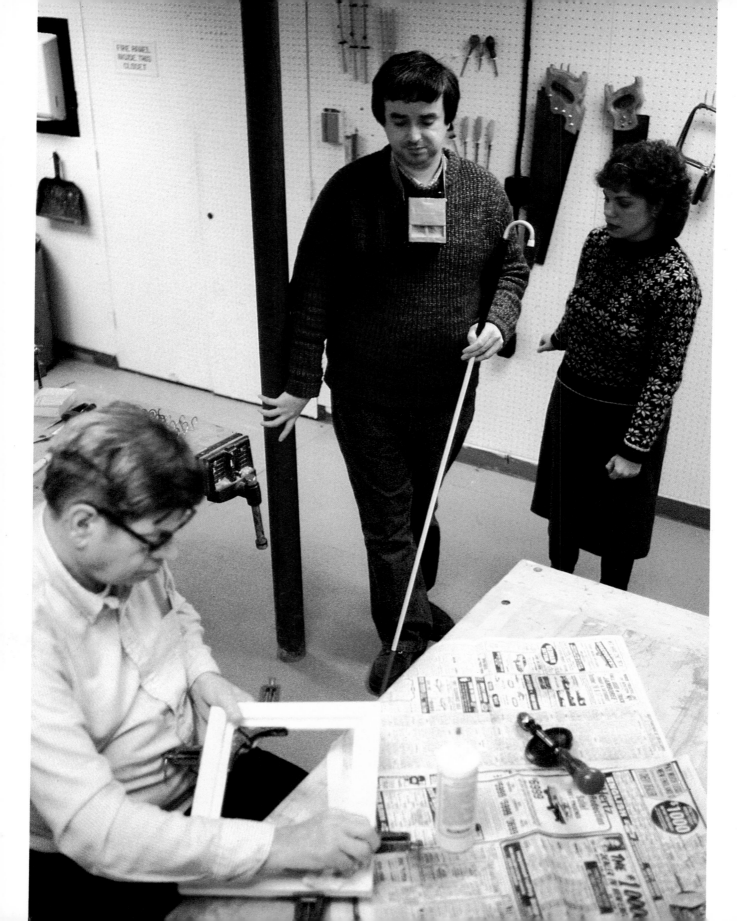

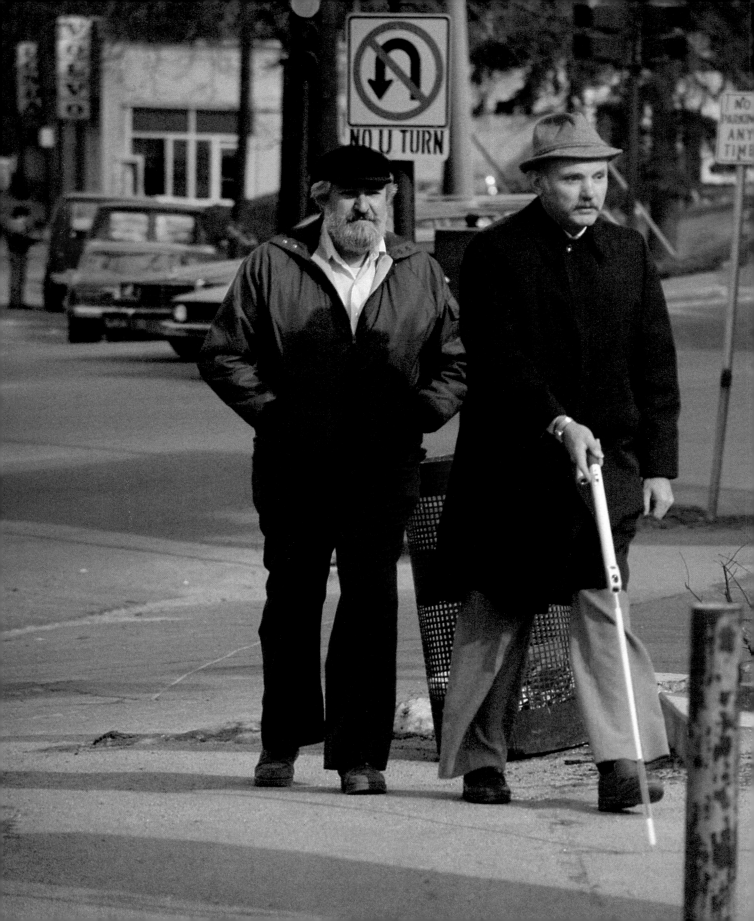

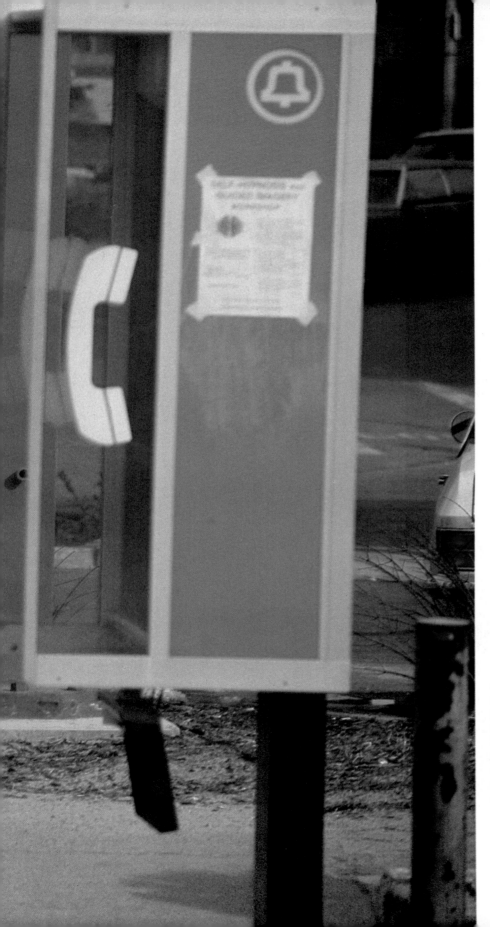

Armed with a Nurion Laser Cane, a man nears an obstacle that an ordinary ground-probing long cane would not detect—a telephone booth raised above the ground. The hazard is sensed by an upward-pointing beam of invisible infrared light, one of three emitted by the cane. The beam bounces off the booth and back to a cell on the cane, setting off a warning tone.

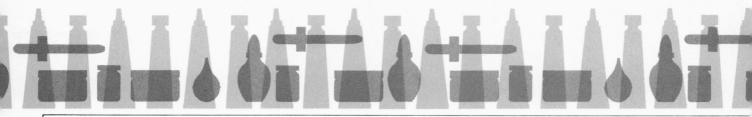

Drugs to correct the senses

Many drugs are available to fight disorders of sight and hearing, but almost none to combat ailments that impair taste, touch and smell. This is due partly to demand and partly to the state of the medical art. Disorders of taste, touch and smell are relatively rare, and their causes and cures remain largely unknown.

The table below, prepared with the help of Christopher S. Conner, Director of the Rocky Mountain Drug Consultation Center, lists the most frequently prescribed medicines effective against ailments of the senses. They are generally topical drugs—applied directly to the affected organ as an ointment, drop or cream. Med-

icines are listed by their chemical names, with trade names underneath. Those containing more than one active ingredient appear with an asterisk; those requiring a prescription are marked Rx.

Heed the following cautions. Pregnant women should consult a physician before taking any drug. Avoid alcohol if you take medicines that cause drowsiness or confusion, and do not drive or operate machinery if you are taking such a drug or one that blurs vision. See a doctor if allergic reactions or serious side effects occur: For example, sore throat, weakness, fever, bruising or bleeding, or prolonged infection may indicate reduced blood counts.

DRUG	Intended effect	Minor side effects	Serious side effects	Special cautions
ACETAZOLAMIDE (Rx) DIAMOX	Controls glaucoma	Appetite loss; nausea; diarrhea; lethargy; depression; frequent urination; dizziness	Kidney stones; increased uric acid in blood; decreased blood-cell counts; fever	Consult doctor before using if you have liver or kidney disease, or if you have gout or have had allergic reactions to sulfa drugs in the past.
ACETIC ACID (Rx) VōSOL OTIC VōSOL HC OTIC*	Cures bacterial infection or fungus in outer-ear canal	Skin irritation or rash	None	Inform doctor if skin irritation or sensitivity develops.
AMPHOTERICIN B (Rx) FUNGIZONE	Cures fungus in outer-ear canal	Itching; skin irritation	Allergic reactions such as skin rash, itching or redness	Use this medicine as directed until it is gone, even if your ear feels better in a few days.
ATROPINE (Rx) **ATROPISOL OPHTHALMIC** **BUFOPTO ATROPINE OPHTHALMIC** **ISOPTO ATROPINE OPHTHALMIC**	Relieves eye inflammation in uveitis and certain kinds of glaucoma	Sensitivity of eyes to light; eye irritation; blurred vision; conjunctivitis	Unsteadiness; flushing; fever; skin rash; mental confusion or hallucinations; unusual tiredness or drowsiness	Consult doctor before using if you have glaucoma. Inform doctor if blurred vision and increased light sensitivity persist for more than two weeks after you discontinue the medicine.
BACITRACIN (Rx) **BACIGUENT OPHTHALMIC**	Cures bacterial eye infections	Burning or stinging eyes	Allergic reactions, such as skin rash, itching or redness	Use this medicine as directed until it is gone, even if your eye feels better in a few days.
BENZOCAINE (Rx) **AMERICAINE-OTIC*** **TYMPAGESIC*** **AURALGAN OTIC***	Relieves pain, swelling and redness in ear infections	Burning or itching in ear	Allergic reactions such as itching, skin rash or difficulty breathing	Consult doctor before using if you are allergic to benzocaine or any local anesthetics, or if you have a perforated eardrum.
CARBACHOL (Rx) **CARBACEL OPHTHALMIC** **ISOPTO CARBACHOL OPHTHALMIC**	Controls glaucoma	Headache; eye pain; blurred vision; eye irritation	Increased perspiration and salivation; frequent urination; shortness of breath; tightness in chest; flushing; diarrhea; vomiting	Consult doctor before using if you have asthma, heart disease, thyroid disease, ulcers or Parkinson's disease.

*Combination drug. Refer also to other active ingredients on label.

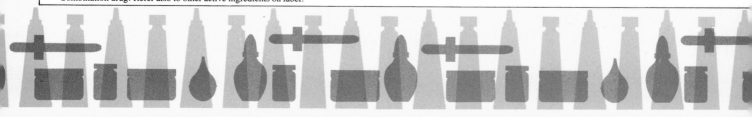

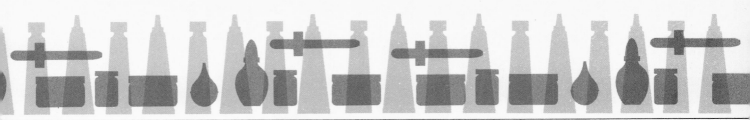

DRUG	Intended effect	Minor side effects	Serious side effects	Special cautions
CARBAMIDE PEROXIDE DEBROX* MURINE EAR DROPS* BENADYNE IMPROVED*	Softens ear wax	None	None	Inform doctor if ear redness, irritation, swelling or pain persists or increases while you are using this medicine.
CHLORAMPHENICOL (OPHTHALMIC) (Rx) CHLOROMYCETIN OPHTHALMIC CHLOROPTIC S.O.P. OPHTHALMIC ECONOCHLOR OPHTHALMIC CHLOROMYXIN OPHTHALMIC*	Cures bacterial eye infections	Stinging or burning eyes	Reduced blood-cell counts after prolonged use; allergic reactions, such as itching, swelling, redness or skin rash	Consult doctor before using if you have blood disorders such as anemia. Inform doctor of fever, sore throat, weakness, bruising or bleeding—signs of reduced blood-cell counts. Take this medicine as directed until it is gone, even if your eye feels better in a few days.
CHLORAMPHENICOL (OTIC) (Rx) CHLOROMYCETIN OTIC	Cures outer-ear infection	Burning ears	Reduced blood-cell counts after prolonged use; allergic reactions, such as itching, redness, swelling or skin rash	Consult doctor before using if you have blood disorders such as anemia. Inform doctor of fever, sore throat, weakness, bruising or bleeding—signs of reduced blood-cell counts. Take this medicine as directed until it is gone, even if your ear feels better in a few days.
CHLOROTHIAZIDE (Rx) DIURIL	Controls Ménière's disease	Lightheadedness when standing; increased urination; sensitivity of skin to light; blurred vision	Potassium deficiency; aggravated diabetes and gout; reduced blood-cell counts; liver disease	Increase intake of potassium-rich foods such as bananas and orange juice. Notify doctor of sore throat, bruising, or bleeding—signs of reduced blood-cell counts.
COLISTIN (OPHTHALMIC) (Rx) COLY-MYCIN S OPHTHALMIC	Cures bacterial eye infections	Burning or stinging eyes	Allergic reactions, such as itching, redness, swelling or skin rash	Use this medicine as directed until it is gone, even if your eye feels better in a few days.
COLISTIN (OTIC) (Rx) COLY-MYCIN S OTIC*	Cures ear infection and relieves associated inflammation	None	Allergic reactions, such as itching, redness, swelling or rash	Consult doctor before using if you have chronic inflammation of the middle ear, a perforated eardrum, or any viral disease. Take this medicine as directed until it is gone, even if your ear feels better in a few days.
CORTISOL (OPHTHALMIC) (Rx) OPTEF HYDROCORTONE OPHTHALMIC NEO-CORTEF*	Relieves eye inflammation	Burning, stinging or watery eyes; dilated pupils	Increased pressure in the eye (glaucoma), vision difficulties, cataract formation, eye infections —all with prolonged use	Consult doctor before using if you have glaucoma or any viral infection of the eye. Inform doctor if no improvement occurs after 5 to 7 days or if the condition worsens. Inform doctor if you see halos around lights— a sign of glaucoma.
CORTISOL (OTIC) (Rx) ORLEX H.C. OTIC* VōSOL HC OTIC* CORTISPORIN OTIC*	Relieves itching and inflammation associated with ear infection	Stinging or burning ears	None	Consult doctor before using if you have a perforated eardrum or viral or fungal conditions of the ear or skin. Avoid prolonged use—inform doctor if the ear condition worsens or if no improvement occurs after 5 to 7 days.
CYCLIZINE MAREZINE	Prevents motion sickness; controls Ménière's disease	Drowsiness; blurred vision; dizziness; dry mouth	Nervousness; insomnia; palpitations; difficulty urinating; skin rash; hallucinations	Consult doctor before taking if you have intestinal obstruction, ulcers, enlarged prostate gland or glaucoma.

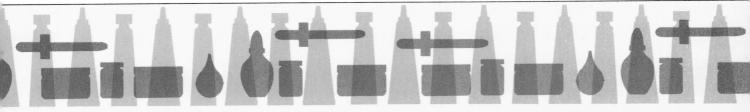

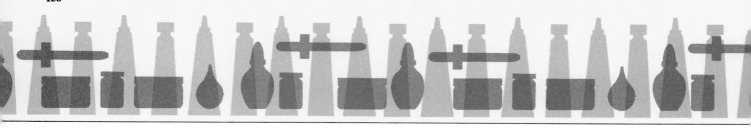

DRUG	Intended effect	Minor side effects	Serious side effects	Special cautions
DEMECARIUM BROMIDE (Rx) HUMORSOL OPHTHALMIC	Controls glaucoma	Headache; eye pain; watery eyes; blurred vision; burning or stinging eyes	Nausea; vomiting; diarrhea; shortness of breath or wheezing; tightness in chest; increased perspiration; weakness or tiredness; frequent urination; confusion; cataracts with prolonged use	Consult doctor before using if you have asthma, a history of retinal detachment, ulcers or cardiovascular disorders. Inform doctor if you are taking this drug, or have taken it recently, before any kind of surgery or work near insecticides.
DEXAMETHASONE (Rx) MAXIDEX OPHTHALMIC DECADRON PHOSPHATE OPHTHALMIC	All effects similar to CORTISOL (OPHTHALMIC)			
DIMENHYDRINATE DRAMAMINE	Prevents motion sickness	Drowsiness; dizziness; dry mouth; nervousness or insomnia, particularly in children	Irregular heartbeat; hallucinations; confusion; delirium; aggravated glaucoma	Consult doctor before taking if you have glaucoma. Take at least 1 hour before travel for maximum effect.
DIPHENHYDRAMINE (Rx) BENADRYL	Prevents and controls motion sickness; controls Ménière's disease	Drowsiness; dizziness; dry mouth; difficulty urinating	Irregular heartbeat; hallucinations; confusion; delirium; aggravated glaucoma	Consult doctor before taking if you have glaucoma, high blood pressure, heart disease or urinary obstruction.
DIPIVEFRIN (Rx) PROPINE	Controls glaucoma	Stinging or burning eyes	Irregular heartbeat; headache; high blood pressure	Consult doctor before using this medicine if you have heart disease or high blood pressure. Inform doctor if you experience irregular heartbeat or headache—signs of absorption of drug from eye.
ECHOTHIOPHATE IODIDE (Rx) PHOSPHOLINE IODIDE ECHODIDE	All effects similar to DEMECARIUM BROMIDE			
EPINEPHRINE (Rx) EPITRATE EPIFRIN EPPY/N EPINAL E-CARPINE*	Controls glaucoma	Headache; stinging, burning or watery eyes	Increased perspiration; tremors; irregular heartbeat; faintness; anxiety or fear; paleness; increased blood pressure	Consult doctor before using if you have high blood pressure, diabetes, thyroid disorders, heart disease or asthma; or if you are taking or have recently taken drugs for depression. Do not use this drug if solution becomes brown or pink or is cloudy. Notify doctor if you are taking this drug before any kind of surgery.
ERYTHROMYCIN (Rx) ILOTYCIN OPHTHALMIC	Cures bacterial eye infections	Burning or stinging eyes	Allergic reactions, such as itching, redness, swelling or skin rash	Use this medicine as directed until it is gone, even if your eye feels better in a few days.
FLUOROMETHOLONE (Rx) FML LIQUIFILM OPHTHALMIC	All effects similar to CORTISOL (OPHTHALMIC)			

*Combination drug. Refer also to other active ingredients on label.

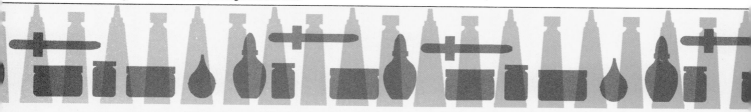

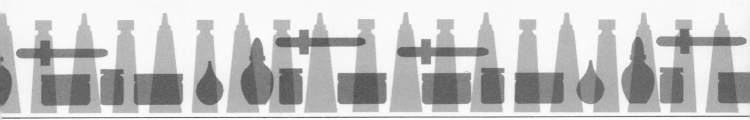

DRUG	Intended effect	Minor side effects	Serious side effects	Special cautions

GENTAMICIN (Rx)
  GARAMYCIN
  OPHTHALMIC
	Cures bacterial eye infections	Burning or stinging eyes	Allergic reactions, such as itching, redness, swelling or skin rash	Use this medicine as directed until it is gone, even if your eye feels better in a few days.

GLYCERIN
  DEBROX*
  E.R.O.*
  MURINE EAR DROPS*
	Softens ear wax	None	None	Consult doctor before using if you have a perforated eardrum.

HYDROCORTISONE	See CORTISOL			

HYDROXYPROPYL
  CELLULOSE
  OPHTHALMIC
  INSERT (Rx)
  LACRISERT
	Relieves dry eyes	Blurred vision; eye irritation; sticky eyelashes	Swollen eyelids; allergic reactions, such as itching, redness, swelling or rash	If one insert is accidentally expelled, another may be placed in the eye. Inform doctor of excessive eye irritation.

IDOXURIDINE (Rx)
  STOXIL
  DENDRID
  HERPLEX LIQUIFILM
	Cures viral eye infections	Eye irritation and watering	Sensitivity of eyes to light; swelling, itching, pain or inflammation of the eye; hazy or blurred vision	Use this medicine until it is gone, even if your eye feels better in a few days. Do not use with boric acid; the combination may cause eye irritation. Notify doctor if the condition worsens or does not improve within a week.

ISOFLUROPHATE (Rx)
  FLOROPRYL
  OPHTHALMIC
	All effects similar to DEMECARIUM BROMIDE			

MECLIZINE
  ANTIVERT (Rx)
  BONINE
	Prevents motion sickness; relieves dizziness; controls Ménière's disease	Drowsiness; dry mouth; blurring of vision	None	Consult doctor before taking if you have asthma, glaucoma, or enlarged prostate gland.

MEDRYSONE (Rx)
  HMS LIQUIFILM
  OPHTHALMIC
	All effects similar to CORTISOL (OPHTHALMIC)			

METHYLCELLULOSE
  MURINE REGULAR
  FORMULA EYE
  DROPS
  METHULOSE
	Relieves eye irritation and dry eyes	None	None	Use only as directed—excess amounts can cause discomfort.

NAPHAZOLINE
  ALBALON LIQUIFILM
  OPHTHALMIC (Rx)
  ALLEREST
	Relieves eye irritation	Stinging eyes; headache	Irregular heartbeat; increased perspiration; increased blood pressure	Consult doctor before using if you have glaucoma, high blood pressure, diabetes or heart disease. Avoid daily use for more than two weeks at a time—psychological dependence may occur.

NATAMYCIN (Rx)
  NATACYN
  MYPROZINE
	Cures fungal eye infections	Stinging or irritated eyes	None	Use this medicine until it is gone, even if your eye feels better in a few days. Inform doctor if the condition worsens or if there is no improvement after a week.

NEOMYCIN SULFATE
  (OPHTHALMIC) (Rx)
  MYCIGUENT
  OPHTHALMIC
	Cures bacterial eye infections	Stinging or burning eyes	Allergic reactions, such as itching, redness, swelling or skin rash	Use this medicine as directed until it is gone, even if your eye feels better in a few days.

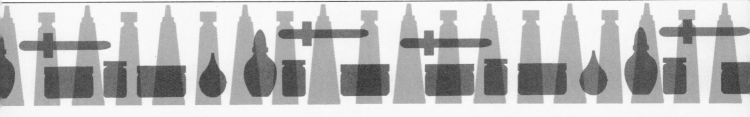

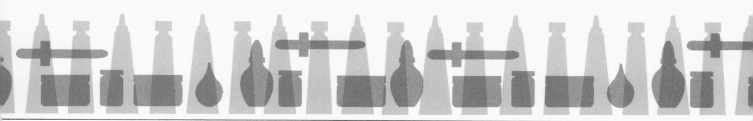

DRUG	Intended effect	Minor side effects	Serious side effects	Special cautions
NEOMYCIN SULFATE (OTIC) (Rx) OTOBIOTIC OTIC CORTISPORIN OTIC* OTOBIONE OTIC*	Cures bacterial infections of outer ear	None	Allergic reactions, such as itching, redness, swelling or skin rash	Consult doctor before using if you have a perforated eardrum. Take this medicine as directed until it is gone, even if your ear feels better within a few days.
PHENYLEPHRINE NEO-SYNEPHRINE OPHTHALMIC (Rx) VASOSULF* (Rx) ISOPTO FRIN ZINCFRIN*	Prescription products control some types of glaucoma; nonprescription products relieve minor eye irritation	Headache; watery or stinging eyes	Tremors; irregular heartbeat; increased perspiration; increased blood pressure	Consult doctor before using if you have diabetes, heart disease or high blood pressure; or if you are taking or have recently taken drugs for depression. Do not use if solution is brownish or cloudy.
PHYSOSTIGMINE (Rx) ESERINE SULFATE OPHTHALMIC ISOPTO ESERINE OPHTHALMIC MIOCEL OPHTHALMIC*	Controls glaucoma	Blurred vision; headache; stinging, burning or watery eyes	Weakness; nausea; diarrhea; vomiting; shortness of breath or wheezing; increased perspiration; irregular heartbeat	Do not use solution if it becomes discolored in any way. Keep solution away from heat and light.
PILOCARPINE (Rx) ISOPTO CARPINE OPHTHALMIC OCUSERT PILO-20 AND -40 OCULAR THERAPEUTIC SYSTEM	Controls glaucoma	Blurred vision; headache; eye irritation	Increased perspiration; nausea; vomiting; diarrhea; tremors; increased salivation	Consult doctor before using if you have any other eye problems or asthma. Keep in refrigerator.
POLYMYXIN B (Rx) AEROSPORIN OTIC LIDOSPORIN OTIC* CORTISPORIN OTIC*	Cures bacterial ear infections	Burning or stinging ears	Allergic reactions, such as itching, redness, swelling or skin rash	Use medicine as directed until it is gone, even if your ear feels better in a few days.
PREDNISOLONE (Rx) ECONOPRED HYDELTRASOL	All effects similar to CORTISOL (OPHTHALMIC)			
PREDNISONE (Rx) DELTASONE ORASONE PARACORT	Relieves symptoms of Bell's palsy	Nausea; indigestion; insomnia; weight gain; muscle cramps; menstrual irregularities	Depression or emotional disturbances; potassium loss; acne; elevated blood pressure; gastric or duodenal ulcer; bone disease; pancreas inflammation; increased pressure in the eye (aggravated glaucoma); impaired immune response	Adhere to a low-salt diet as outlined by your physician. Inform doctor of black tarry stools or persistent stomach pain—signs of bleeding from the stomach or intestine. Do not discontinue abruptly after prolonged use—adverse reactions can occur, such as fever, weakness and dangerous decreases in blood pressure. Do not submit to any vaccinations or skin tests without consulting your doctor.
SCOPOLAMINE (OPHTHALMIC) (Rx) ISOPTO HYOSCINE OPHTHALMIC	All effects similar to ATROPINE			

*Combination drug. Refer also to other active ingredients on label.

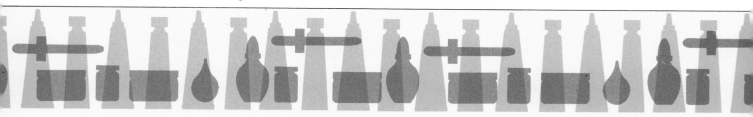

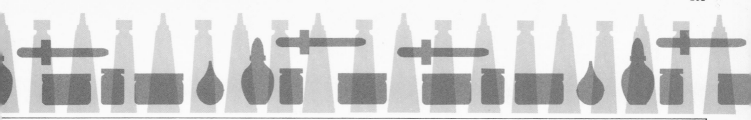

DRUG	Intended effect	Minor side effects	Serious side effects	Special cautions
SCOPOLAMINE (TOPICAL) (Rx) TRANSDERM-V	Prevents motion sickness	Dry mouth; drowsiness; blurred vision	Disorientation; restlessness; mental confusion; hallucinations	Consult doctor before using if you have glaucoma or intestinal or urinary obstruction. Apply only to the skin behind the ear. Wash hands and dry thoroughly before and after applying this medicine. Apply several hours before travel.
SULFACETAMIDE (Rx) BLEPH-10 LIQUIFILM SODIUM SULAMYD VASOSULF* CETAMIDE	Cures eye infections	Stinging or burning eyes	Allergic reactions, such as itching, redness, swelling or skin rash	Consult doctor before using if you have an allergy to diuretics, such as hydrochlorothiazide or furosemide, or to sulfa drugs. Use this medicine as directed until it is gone, even if your eye feels better in a few days.
SULFISOXAZOLE DIOLAMINE (Rx) GANTRISIN	All effects similar to SULFACETAMIDE			
TETRAHYDROZOLINE VISINE MURINE PLUS	All effects similar to NAPHAZOLINE			
TETRACYCLINE (Rx) ACHROMYCIN OPHTHALMIC	Cures eye infections	Burning or stinging eyes	None	Use this medicine as directed until it is gone, even if your eye feels better in a few days. Inform doctor if the condition worsens or if no improvement occurs within a week.
THIMEROSAL MERTHIOLATE OPHTHALMIC	Cures conjunctivitis and prevents infection following removal of foreign bodies	Stinging or burning eyes	Allergic reactions, such as redness, itching, swelling or skin rash	Consult doctor before using if you have an allergy to mercury.
TIMOLOL MALEATE (Rx) TIMOPTIC	Controls glaucoma	Eye irritation	Slow heartbeat; reduced blood pressure; difficulty breathing; mental disturbances, including confusion and depression	Consult doctor before using if you have irregular heartbeat, asthma, lung disease, heart disease or high blood pressure.
TRIETHANOLAMINE POLYPEPTIDE OLEATE-CONDENSATE (Rx) CERUMENEX	Dissolves ear wax	Ear irritation	Skin rash	Consult doctor before using if you have a perforated eardrum or an inflammation of the middle ear.
TRIFLURIDINE (Rx) VIROPTIC	Cures viral eye infections	Burning or stinging eyes; inflammation or swelling of eyelids	Allergic reactions, such as redness, itching or skin rash; increased pressure in the eye; cornea irritation or damage	Use this medicine as directed until it is gone, even if your eye feels better in a few days. Notify doctor if the condition worsens or if no improvement occurs within a week.
VIDARABINE (Rx) VIRA-A	Cures viral eye infections	Stinging or watery eyes; irritated eyes	Cornea inflammation; eye pain; sensitivity of eyes to light; allergic reactions, such as itching, redness, swelling or skin rash	Use this medicine as directed until it is gone, even if your eye feels better in a few days. Notify doctor if the condition worsens or if improvement is not seen within a week.

An encyclopedia of symptoms

Almost everyone occasionally suffers at least a temporary impairment of one of the senses, perhaps no more serious than a common cold's interference with the ability to smell and taste. Although defects in any of the senses are real handicaps, problems with sight or hearing are of the greatest. These senses, too, are often affected by symptoms of no consequence; occasionally seeing spots before your eyes or hearing ringing in your ears means nothing in most cases. But the very same effects, if they are recurrent or persistent, can be early warnings of serious disease.

It is important to understand which symptoms mean what, so that you can know when to ignore them, when to treat them yourself and when to consult a doctor. The symptoms of the most common disorders of the senses are described below, listed alphabetically by conditions that can be felt or seen. The disorder associated with each symptom—or each group of symptoms—is named in small capital letters.

Astigmatism. *See BLURRED VISION*

Bloodshot eyes. *See RED EYES*

BLURRED VISION. The inability to bring objects into focus is a common complaint. It can be the result of a blow to the eye or head, of excessive alcohol consumption or of a problem with the eyes. Blurred or fuzzy vision always should be reported to an eye doctor, for it can indicate or presage any of several serious eye ailments (see DIMMING VISION, EYE PAIN). Far more often, however, blurred or fuzzy vision suggests an easily correctable REFRACTIVE ERROR, an inability of the eye to focus light on the retina.

If distant objects are blurred or fuzzy but near objects are seen clearly, the problem may be MYOPIA, or nearsightedness, in which images are brought to a focus in front of the retina because the eyeball is unusually long from front to back. A concave corrective lens will solve the problem.

If near objects are blurred but distant objects are clear, the problem may be HYPEROPIA, or farsightedness, in which images are brought to a focus behind the retina because the eyeball is unusually short from front to back. A convex corrective lens will solve the problem. Similar blurring of near vision comes from PRESBYOPIA, a condition of aging in which the eye lenses lose their elasticity and so cannot change shape to focus on objects close up. Most people first notice the condition when they are in their forties. As with ordinary hyperopia, a convex corrective lens will solve the problem.

If near and distant objects are blurred, the problem may be ASTIGMATISM, irregular curvature of the corneas. Some objects may be in perfect focus while others, at the same distance, are not. Corrective lenses ground so that they compensate for the irregularities normally solve the problem.

● **Blurred vision that persists after repeated efforts to correct it with spectacles or contact lenses** suggests a vision disorder requiring intensive medical investigation.

If persistent focusing difficulty is accompanied by vision that is misty or cloudy overall, the cause may be a CATARACT, a clouding of the eye lens. This condition usually occurs in people over 50 and progressively dims vision; early symptoms are halos around lights and difficulty driving against oncoming headlights at night. Consult an eye doctor within a few days.

● **Blurred vision that occurs suddenly in a red, painful eye and that is accompanied by nausea and vomiting** may suggest ACUTE GLAUCOMA, a disease characterized by a sudden rise in pressure of the fluid inside the eyeball. This disorder usually affects people over 40. Consult an eye doctor immediately.

● **Blurred vision occurring with eye redness and discharge** may suggest CONJUNCTIVITIS, an inflammation of the whites of the eyes and the undersides of the eyelids. Such blurring is caused by the discharge and should be relieved temporarily by blinking. The ailment normally disappears by itself, but medical treatment can speed the process. See a doctor if no improvement occurs in two days.

● **Blurred vision that occurs with a red, painful eye and sensitivity to light** may suggest KERATITIS, inflammation of the cornea. Consult a physician within several hours.

BURNING SENSATIONS. *See TOUCH CHANGES*

Clogged ears. This common sensation ordinarily is accompanied by a diminished ability to hear and may be caused by nothing more than a sudden change in barometric pressure, such as occurs in an elevator or airplane. You can usually return hearing to normal by swallowing repeatedly or by attempting to exhale gently through the nose while at the same time holding it tightly closed. Other frequent causes of ear blockage are COMMON COLD and ALLERGIC RHINITIS, sensitivity to pollen or environmental chemicals. In such cases, the tube between the ears and the nose becomes swollen and partially obstructed; changes in barometric pressure can worsen such blockage, making it painful and more difficult to relieve. Take decongestant tablets or use nasal sprays to reduce tissue inflammation and help unclog the ears. In most instances, however, ear blockage results from the accumulation of natural body substances in ear passages.

● **Ear blockage and hearing loss** may be caused by impacted wax in the outer-ear canal. Such an occurrence suggests either an abnormally shaped ear canal or, more commonly, that the wax has been pushed into the canal during ineffective attempts to remove it. The best way to clear the ears of wax is to irrigate them with warm water *(page 40)*. Consult a physician if symptoms persist or worsen.

● **Ear blockage can accompany any of several infections** that make fluids accumulate in the middle or outer ear.

If a clogged ear is associated with ear pain, itching and tenderness on touching the ear, or is accompanied by a discharge that is either watery or thick and foul-smelling, the cause may be OTITIS EXTERNA, an infection of the outer-ear canal. Consult a physician within 24 hours.

If a clogged ear is associated with ear pain, fever and hearing loss in the affected ear, it may indicate OTITIS MEDIA, an infected middle ear. Consult a physician within several hours.

● **A sensation of fullness in one ear that is associated with persistent ringing in the ear,** headache and recurrent attacks of severe dizziness may suggest MÉNIÈRE'S DISEASE, an accumulation of fluid in the parts of the inner ear that register balance and sound. The condition primarily affects middle-aged men. Consult a physician within a few days, or sooner if symptoms are severe.

CLOUDY VISION. This complaint is subtly different from the blurred or fuzzy vision brought on by REFRACTIVE ERRORS (see BLURRED VISION). Objects seem in focus but are obscured by haze. Consult an eye doctor—but first make sure you cannot eliminate the haze simply by cleaning your eyeglasses.

● **Cloudy vision that occurs in a person over 50** may suggest a CATARACT, loss of transparency of the eye's lens because of rearrangements in lens molecules. Halos may be seen around lights; driving may be difficult at night, as light from headlights scatters into a bright fog. Some victims report greater difficulty seeing in bright daylight. Consult an eye doctor within several days.

COLOR BLINDNESS. The inability to distinguish certain colors is a relatively rare, inherited condition; it affects less than 10 per cent of the population, mostly men, and is caused by a defect of the cones, the light-sensitive cells in the retina that distinguish colors. Most victims suffer from either red or green color blindness; they are likely to confuse red, orange, yellow and yellow-green, or to see the red or the green shades as yellow. Almost no one is totally colorblind, seeing only shades of light and dark. There is no treatment for color blindness, and it is generally a minor handicap—except for children in school, where an inability to identify colors may occasionally interfere with studies. If color blindness is suspected, the child should be examined by an eye doctor so that necessary assistance can be given in schoolwork.

CROSS-EYES. *See UNCOORDINATED EYES*

Deafness. *See HEARING LOSS*

DIMMING VISION. Unlike the common REFRACTIVE ERRORS that merely blur the view (see BLURRED VISION), dimming vision is characterized by a loss of sight. It can be caused by injury or disease. When injury is at fault, the vision loss usually is sudden, the cause obvious, and the proper response equally so—an immediate trip to the hospital. Dimming vision brought on by disease, however, can occur suddenly or gradually, in one or both eyes, at the center of vision or at the sides. It can occur with or without pain, with accompanying symptoms or by itself. Its origins can be in structures at the front of the eye, or in the retina, which is at the back of the eye, or in the nerves that lead to the brain. Any episode of dim vision should be reported to an eye doctor.

● **Dimming vision that occurs gradually and painlessly in a person over 50 and is marked in its early stages by cloudy vision** or by a sensation of looking through a waterfall may suggest a CATARACT, a clouding of the lens. It generally is noticed first in one eye and may develop over several years. Vision usually is worse at night, but some victims report greater difficulty seeing in bright light. Halos may appear around lights. Dimming vision may have been preceded by frequent changes of prescription in corrective lenses. Consult an eye doctor within several days.

● **Dimming vision that occurs gradually and painlessly in a person over 40 and is marked by loss of side vision or by halos around lights** may suggest CHRONIC GLAUCOMA, a disorder characterized by a gradual rise in pressure of the fluid inside the eyeball. Consult an eye doctor within a day. Although peripheral vision is the first to suffer, this disorder eventually can destroy central vision and cause total blindness. Be on particular guard if relatives have had it: The disease runs in families.

● **Dimming vision that comes on gradually and painlessly in someone who has diabetes,** a disorder of the body's sugar- and starch-processing system, may be a symptom of DIABETIC RETINOPATHY, in which blood-vessel damage brought on by diabetes leads to degeneration of the retina. The dimming of vision may be preceded by seeing spots, stars or ''floaters'' across the field of vision. Consult an eye doctor who specializes in treating this condition, and do so within a day.

● **Dimming vision that occurs gradually and painlessly in an elderly person and that primarily affects central vision** may suggest MACULAR DEGENERATION, a phenomenon of aging in which the portion of the retina responsible for sharp central vision, the macula, deteriorates as blood-vessel changes diminish nourishment delivered to the eye cells. Central vision may be fuzzy and dim at first, then nonexistent. This condition is essentially untreatable, but consult a physician within a day or so to rule out other ailments.

● **Dimming vision that occurs suddenly and painlessly and afflicts one or both eyes** can indicate any of several conditions, all of which demand immediate medical attention.

If dimmed vision occurs suddenly and painlessly in one eye in an elderly person, the cause may be RETINAL ARTERY OCCLUSION, blockage of the main artery serving the retina. Such blockage may be the result of a blood clot or of the hardening of the artery with fatty deposits called atherosclerotic placques.

If dimmed vision occurs suddenly and painlessly in one eye and produces the sensation of a curtain being drawn across the affected eye, the cause may be a RETINAL DETACHMENT, separation of the retina from its underlying layers at the back of the eye. The vision loss may follow a blow to the head or eye. Flashing lights or a shower of spots across the visual field may precede the vision loss.

If dimmed vision occurs suddenly and painlessly in one or both eyes and is associated with nausea, vomiting, headache, dizziness and abdominal pain, the problem could be poisoning by wood alcohol or badly distilled home-brewed liquor.

● **Dimmed vision that occurs suddenly and is accompanied by eye pain** demands immediate attention: Go to a hospital emergency room without delay.

If suddenly and severely dimmed vision in one or both eyes is associated with a red, severely painful eye as well as with nausea and vomiting, the cause may be ACUTE GLAUCOMA, increased pressure of the fluid inside the eyeball caused by excess fluid in the eye. Such episodes occasionally are preceded by periods of slightly diminished vision, by visual disturbances such as halos around lights or by pain in the eye.

If suddenly and severely dimmed vision is associated with a red, painful eye and marked sensitivity to light, it may indicate KERATITIS, inflammation of the cornea, or UVEITIS, inflammation of the iris. Such vision loss may be preceded by blurred vision or by visual disturbances such as seeing halos around lights.

If suddenly and severely dimmed vision is associated with pain on eye movement or on touching the eye, the cause may be OPTIC NEURITIS, inflammation of the eye's nerve. Although symptoms may pass, they can be an early sign of MULTIPLE SCLEROSIS, a nerve disorder also causing difficulty with speech and movement.

DIZZINESS. Dizziness encompasses several different sensations —lightheadedness, unsteadiness, feelings of faintness or a swaying or giddy feeling. Many drugs—including some oral contraceptives, tranquilizers, antidepressants, antihistamines and diuretics —can cause dizziness. Other frequent causes of dizziness are simple REFRACTIVE ERRORS (see BLURRED VISION) and, sometimes, the eye-muscle weakness of STRABISMUS (see UNCOORDINATED EYES).

Vertigo is a severe form of dizziness in which there are feelings that the body is whirling or rotating or that the room is spinning. This indicates a major disturbance of the balance mechanism in the inner ear and is almost always accompanied by nausea, vomiting and pale, sweaty skin.

● **Dizziness that occurs suddenly, upon arising from a sitting or lying position,** most often indicates a temporary reduction in blood flow to the brain. Vision may be reduced or stars or spots may be seen. The problem is particularly common after prolonged bed rest and among elderly individuals. If episodes of dizziness are infrequent, they are probably nothing to worry about, but consult a physician if they persist or recur.

● **Dizziness that occurs while traveling—usually in a car or on a boat—and that is accompanied by nausea or vomiting** or by pale or clammy skin may suggest MOTION SICKNESS, a disturbance of the balance mechanism in the inner ear. If you are prone to motion sickness, take a preventive drug *(page 22)* before you travel; while traveling, fix your eyes on the horizon and open some windows if possible.

● **Dizziness or giddiness that occurs suddenly, along with rapid shallow breathing, increased heart rate, and sweating** may indicate an ANXIETY ATTACK, a psychosomatic problem in which rapid breathing decreases the amount of carbon dioxide in the blood. Breathe into a paper bag in order to build up carbon dioxide in your bloodstream and break the attack. Consult a physician immediately if symptoms persist.

● **Dizziness that is mild but persistent and that is accompanied by ringing in the ear or hearing loss** may be an indication of ACOUSTIC NEUROMA, a brain tumor located on the nerve to the ear. Persistent headache may occur as well. Consult a physician within the next several days.

● **Vertigo can have a variety of causes,** and should always be investigated by a physician.

If vertigo is recurrent and is associated with hearing loss or ringing or fullness in the ear, it may suggest MÉNIÈRE'S DISEASE, an accumulation of fluid in the parts of the inner ear that register balance and sound. It primarily affects middle-aged men. Consult a physician within several days.

If vertigo occurs suddenly and is associated with ringing in the ears and a staggering gait, it may indicate ACUTE LABYRINTHITIS, an inflammation of the inner ear often caused by a viral infection. Consult a physician within several hours.

DOUBLE VISION. This unpleasant symptom, called diplopia by doctors, can be brought about by fatigue, a blow to the head, an injury to the eye or the excessive consumption of alcohol or drugs. Double vision usually passes quickly, but if it is severe or persists, bring it to the attention of an eye doctor. Double vision occasionally is the result of a chronic disorder of the eyes themselves, usually an inability of the eyes to work together and focus simultaneously on the same object.

● **Double vision that occurs in a person whose eyes turn abnormally** inward (cross-eye), outward (walleye) or upward (hypertropia), either together or independently of each other, usually suggests STRABISMUS, an imbalance in the muscles that control eye movement. The condition is most common in children. Double vision may be severe or mild, constant or intermittent. In some cases of strabismus, double vision does not occur at all, because the brain in effect accepts the nerve signals from only one eye, and overrides the nerve signals from the other. But this unconscious adaptation can lead to blindness in that eye as the brain refuses altogether to respond to its signals. Consult a physician within several days. Eye exercises in many cases can correct the problem; so can special glasses designed to strengthen eye muscles that are weak. Surgery helps in severe cases.

● **Double vision and other vision disturbances, such as focusing difficulty, that occur with or immediately after nausea, vomiting, abdominal cramps and diarrhea** may suggest BOTULISM, a potentially fatal food poisoning that is caused by the Clostridium bacterium. There may also be difficulty swallowing or speaking. This medical emergency demands immediate attention. Go to a hospital emergency room without delay.

DRY EYES. Exposure to a dry or smoke-filled environment often produces irritated, bloodshot eyes that may feel dry or scratchy. Rest, go to an area with cleaner air or ask people to stop smoking. Use any over-the-counter eye drops that seem to soothe your eyes. Persistently dry eyes that have a sandy, gritty or burning feeling, usually worse during the day and better on awakening, are another matter and should receive a doctor's attention.

● **Persistently dry eyes that may or may not be bloodshot usually** suggest KERATOCONJUNCTIVITIS SICCA; the name simply means drying of the outer surface of the eyeball. Sensitivity to light may occur as well. Use eye drops containing methyl-cellulose, often referred to as artificial tears. Consult a physician within several days if symptoms do not improve; other, more serious disorders can bring the same symptoms.

● **Persistently dry, tearless eyes that are associated with dryness of the nose, mouth, throat or vagina** may suggest SJÖGREN'S SYNDROME, a connective-tissue disease of middle-aged women. Arthritis or joint pain may accompany this disorder. Consult a physician within a few days.

EARACHE. Pain in the ears is most common in childhood but can occur later in life. True pain should be distinguished from the sensation of a clogged ear (see CLOGGED EARS). Yet ear pain may occur simultaneously with such a sensation of fullness or blockage because of excess secretions or swollen tissues in the outer-ear canal or in the middle ear.

● **Earache that occurs with itching and visible redness in the ear** as well as severe pain on moving the outer ear may suggest OTITIS EXTERNA, an infection in the outer-ear canal. This condition can result from inadequate drying of the ear after swimming or bathing. More often it follows overzealous attempts to clean the outer-ear canal. Additional symptoms can include a crusty, scaly or watery discharge from the ear. Consult a physician within 24 hours, sooner if pain is severe.

● **Earache that occurs with a sensation of fullness and with hearing loss and fever** may indicate OTITIS MEDIA, an infection of the middle ear. The condition often is preceded or accompanied by an upper-respiratory infection (a common cold or influenza, say) and a stuffy nose, particularly in young children. Pain may be severe. It may be relieved suddenly when a thick, yellow discharge exudes from the ear. This event shows that there has been a tear in the middle-ear membrane, or eardrum, caused by the build-up of pus behind it. In most cases the perforated eardrum will heal, and hearing will return to normal. Whether or not there is discharge, consult a physician about a middle-ear ache within several hours; middle-ear infections remain an important cause of deafness, although most can be cured quickly with antibiotics.

● **Earache can be caused by pain that is referred** from disorders outside the ear.

If ear pain is accompanied by fever and tenderness over the cheek, the cause may be either a tooth infection or SINUSITIS, an infection of the sensitive air pockets in the bones of the cheek. Consult a physician within 24 hours. In the meantime, take aspirin and apply hot compresses to relieve the pain.

If ear pain is associated with pain on chewing or on opening the jaw widely, these symptoms may point to TEMPOROMANDIBULAR JOINT SUBLUXATION, improper alignment of the jaw joint. There may be clicking or locking of the jaw, and you may feel tenderness on touching the edge of the cheek, just in front of the ear. Consult a physician within several days.

EAR DISCHARGE. The outer-ear canal normally produces small particles of wax that can be removed by gentle cleaning or irrigation with warm water *(page 40)*. Discharge of fluid or other material from the ear demands medical attention.

● **Watery or blood-tinged fluid that flows from the ear after a head injury** may suggest a BASAL SKULL FRACTURE, a break in the bone that surrounds the ear. Get medical attention immediately.

• **Watery discharge from an ear that has been itchy or otherwise irritated** may indicate OTITIS EXTERNA, an infection of the outer-ear canal. The canal may be red or have crusty scales, and the discharge, though usually watery, can be thick and foul-smelling. There may be a sensation of ear blockage, earache or severe pain on moving or touching the outer ear. Consult a physician within 24 hours, or sooner if symptoms are severe.

• **Thick, yellow ear discharge that occurs suddenly and relieves a painful, clogged ear** may indicate a perforated eardrum. Such breakage normally occurs when pus from a middle-ear infection builds to an excessive degree. The discharge may be slightly blood-tinged. There may be fever and hearing loss in the affected ear. Consult a physician within a few hours.

• **Ear discharge that is scant in amount but that has a distinctly foul odor,** and that is not accompanied by an earache, may be a symptom of CHOLESTEATOMA, an abnormal growth of skinlike tissue inside the middle ear, often resulting from recurrent ear infections. There can be some hearing loss in the affected ear. Consult a physician within several days.

EYELID INFLAMMATION. The edges of the eyelids are prone to inflammation. The condition often begins in childhood but can continue through later life.

If the edges of the eyelids are red and lined by fine, greasy, dandruff-like flakes or scales, the problem may be BLEPHARITIS, a skin infection that is in many cases accompanied by dandruff of the scalp, eyebrows, nose or ears. Surrounding the base of the lashes may be crusty material that is sticky and difficult to remove. Prescription drugs sometimes are needed to clear up such an infection; consult a physician if the inflammation does not begin to go away after several days.

EYELID SWELLING. The eyelids are particularly prone to conditions that produce swelling. Such swelling can occur suddenly in one or both eyes, with or without pain or itching.

• **Painless swelling in both eyes,** which may occur suddenly or develop gradually, is often an indication of excess body fluid. Hands, feet or legs may also swell. One frequent cause in women is MENSTRUAL FLUID RETENTION, the accumulation of excess water in the body during the week prior to the menses. The symptom may also suggest NEPHROTIC SYNDROME, a kidney disease marked by severe protein loss and generalized swelling. Consult a physician if persistent swelling occurs without explanation.

• **Swelling of one eyelid that occurs suddenly with some pain and itching** may indicate an insect bite. The bite itself may not have been felt. Apply ice and take antihistamines; the swelling is an allergic reaction. Consult a physician if symptoms are severe or persistent or if there is any loss or impairment of vision.

• **Swelling of one eyelid with a localized red, painful, tender lump** may indicate a HORDEOLUM, a common sty. This condition—an infection of an eyelid gland—can occur on either the outer or the inner surface of the eyelid. Apply warm compresses for 10 to 15 minutes, four times a day. Consult a physician if symptoms do not begin to clear up within a few days.

If a small lump in the eyelid is not accompanied by pain, redness or tenderness, it may be a CHALAZION, an inflamed nodule in an eyelid gland. Apply warm compresses for 10 to 15 minutes, four times a day. Consult a physician if the lump does not disappear within two weeks.

• **Painful swelling that is primarily confined to the inner corner of the eye** may indicate ACUTE DACRYOCYSTITIS, an infected tear gland. There may be excess tearing and a thick discharge as well. Apply hot compresses for 10 to 15 minutes, four times a day, and consult a physician within 24 hours.

EYELID TWITCHING. This common condition almost always is the result of fatigue or overuse of the eyes. The best cure is to get extra rest and to rest your eyes periodically while doing close work. Report persistent eyelid twitching to your doctor.

EYE PAIN. Pain in and around the eyes can indicate a variety of disorders involving the surface of the eyes, its inner structures and the surrounding tissues of the face and brain. The problem may be TENSION HEADACHE, MIGRAINE HEADACHE or CLUSTER HEADACHE (see HEAD PAIN), but the most common cause of eye pain is some foreign material, such as an eyelash or a speck of dirt, lodging on the outer surface of the eye. You can usually remove such an object by pulling the upper eyelid down and allowing the lower eyelashes to brush the material away or by flushing the eye with water. If pain persists or is accompanied by other disturbing visual effects, consult an eye doctor.

• **Pain that persists after the eye has been flushed** usually indicates either an embedded particle or a CORNEAL ABRASION, a scratch on the cornea, the transparent membrane that covers the iris and lens. Do not rub the eye; keep it closed and consult a physician within a few hours.

• **Eye pain that occurs after prolonged reading or close work** may suggest a REFRACTIVE ERROR, improper focusing of light on the retina. Such eyestrain may be accompanied by blurred vision, but this telltale sign of focusing difficulty need not occur. Rest your eyes periodically from close work or prolonged reading by closing them briefly or focusing them on a distant object. Make sure you have adequate light for the task at hand. Consult an eye doctor if the discomfort persists; corrective lenses usually solve the problem.

• **Eye pain that occurs with sudden visual impairment** indicates a serious disorder requiring immediate treatment.

If severe eye pain occurs suddenly and is associated with redness and blurred vision, or with nausea and vomiting, the cause may be ACUTE GLAUCOMA, increased pressure on the retina caused by excess fluid inside the eyeball. It is occasionally preceded by warnings that many people ignore—episodes of brief, temporary eye pain and blurred vision, occurring particularly in darkened rooms such as theaters, where the pupil must dilate. Consult a physician immediately.

If pain on eye movement occurs suddenly and is associated with either blurred, decreased or lost vision, the cause may be OPTIC NEURITIS, inflammation of the optic nerve. Consult a physician within several hours if symptoms do not pass. If symptoms disappear, you can wait until the next day. OPTIC NEURITIS is often an early sign of MULTIPLE SCLEROSIS, a progressive nerve disease that also causes difficulty with speech and movement.

If eye pain on exposure to light is associated with cloudy or blurred vision, the cause may be either KERATITIS, infection of the cornea, or UVEITIS, infection of the iris. Redness or excess secretions in the eye as well as halos around lights may occur. Consult a physician immediately.

If eye pain and sensitivity to light follow exposure to ultraviolet light—usually from sunlamps, welding torches or sunlight reflected off snow or water—the cause may be SNOW BLINDNESS, called ULTRAVIOLET KERATITIS, the inflammation of the cornea by ultraviolet rays. There may be excess watering of the eyes and the sensation of a foreign body, grit or sand in the eyes. Symptoms frequently occur six to nine hours after exposure. The condition will subside by itself in two to three days. Medical treatment can ease pain but cannot speed healing.

FARSIGHTEDNESS. *See BLURRED VISION*

HEAD PAIN.
Head pain often is a temporary response to the stresses of daily life. Yet because so many of the sensory organs are located in the head, many people believe that head pain positively suggests a problem with a sense organ, particularly the eyes. It rarely does. For example, pain or tightness over the brow, around the eyes and forehead may be the product of eyestrain—fatigue of the eyes caused by prolonged close work in glaring or dim light—but it is more commonly caused by TENSION HEADACHE, muscle contraction due to stress. Rest, relax and take aspirin to relieve pain. In some cases, however, such frontal head pain can suggest REFRAC-

TIVE ERROR, improper light focusing by the eyes. Consult a physician if such symptoms recur frequently.

• **Sharp, severe head pain that is centered around one red, tearful eye** and that is associated with a clogged nostril and flushed skin on that side of the face may suggest CLUSTER HEADACHE. This condition usually afflicts adult men. Consult a physician within a day, sooner if pain is severe.

• **Throbbing pain on one side of the head** may suggest one of the two forms of MIGRAINE HEADACHE.

If throbbing, one-sided head pain is accompanied by nausea and vomiting and by uncomfortable sensitivity to light and noise, the cause may be COMMON MIGRAINE HEADACHE. Consult a physician so that treatment can be started.

If throbbing, one-sided head pain is preceded by a 15- to 30-minute period of unusual visual disturbances, language disturbances or unusual sensations such as tingling or numbness of the hands, the cause may be CLASSIC MIGRAINE HEADACHE. Consult a physician so that treatment can be started.

HEARING LOSS. Hearing loss can occur suddenly or gradually, in one or both ears, and at any age. When sudden, it may be accompanied by a sensation of clogged or blocked ears. This common experience is often the result of changes in barometric pressure or of wax impacted in the outer-ear canal (see CLOGGED EARS). Such conditions need not cause concern unless they are annoyingly frequent or unusually disturbing. Other conditions that produce hearing loss, however, demand a doctor's attention.

• **Progressive hearing loss that develops gradually in an older individual** may indicate PRESBYCUSIS, a stiffening and deterioration of sound receptors in the ear, resulting from aging. Consult a physician within several days.

• **Progressive hearing loss that begins in middle life** may be a symptom of OTOSCLEROSIS, a hereditary disorder in which the stapes, one of the small bones in the middle ear, becomes immobilized and is unable to transmit sound vibrations. Consult a physician within several days.

• **Temporary hearing loss that is accompanied by earache, a feeling of fullness in the ear or fever** may indicate OTITIS MEDIA, an infection of the middle ear. A thick discharge from the ear can occur suddenly, indicating a perforated eardrum, which may relieve the pain but worsen the hearing loss. Such infections, when neglected, are a common cause of permanent deafness; consult a physician within several hours.

• **Sudden hearing loss that is accompanied by a feeling of fullness in the ear or by an unnatural echoing** of the spoken voice may suggest SEROUS OTITIS MEDIA, an accumulation of sterile fluid in the middle ear. This often occurs in children who suffer recurrent earaches or allergies. Consult a physician within several days.

● **Hearing loss that gets progressively worse and is accompanied by ringing in the ear as well as recurring attacks of severe dizziness** may suggest MÉNIÈRE'S DISEASE, a disorder of the inner ear that primarily affects adult men. Attacks of dizziness, called vertigo, are often so severe as to cause nausea, vomiting and profuse sweating. Consult a physician within several days, sooner if symptoms are severe.

If progressive hearing loss in one ear is associated with ringing in the ear and with mild episodes of dizziness, the problem may be ACOUSTIC NEUROMA, a tumor on the nerve to the ear. Symptoms may progress slowly for several years before becoming noticeably uncomfortable. Consult a physician within a few days.

ITCHY EYES. Itchy, watery eyes almost always indicate ALLERGIC CONJUNCTIVITIS, sensitivity of the undersides of the eyelids and the whites of the eyes to pollens or chemicals in the environment. Allergic conjunctivitis can be the result of HAY FEVER, the seasonal allergy to ragweed pollen that usually causes a runny nose as well as itchy, watery eyes. Another, even more common cause of eye allergy is exposure to hair spray and eye make-up. Symptoms will abate only after the offending chemicals have been removed. Take antihistamines to reduce itching and consult a physician if symptoms persist or worsen.

LAZY EYES. *See UNCOORDINATED EYES*

MOTION SICKNESS. *See DIZZINESS*

NEARSIGHTEDNESS. *See BLURRED VISION*

NIGHT BLINDNESS. Difficulty seeing at night is a frequent complaint. It can be caused by any number of serious and minor eye disorders, from CATARACTS to simple REFRACTIVE ERRORS (see BLURRED VISION, DIMMING VISION). Severely impaired or nonexistent nighttime vision is another, far more serious matter. The problem always originates in the retina's rods, the cells near the edge of the retina that respond to dim light.

● **Night blindness may be brought on by a deficiency of vitamin A.** (Vitamin A is necessary for the production of retinal pigments whose reaction to light initiates the nerve signals of sight.) This condition is quite rare and generally affects males under the age of 20. Consult a physician within a few days.

● **Night blindness that is first noticed in adolescence or young adulthood,** and that is associated with a slow, general deterioration of vision, may suggest RETINITIS PIGMENTOSA, a rare, inherited disorder in which the light-sensitive cells of the retina degenerate. The rods, which provide vision in dim light, deteriorate first, followed months or years later by the cones, the less-sensitive cells in the center that see sharply. There is no cure; blindness is an almost inevitable outcome.

NUMBNESS. *See TOUCH CHANGES*

RED EYES. Redness is the most common of all eye symptoms. It usually is caused by lack of sleep, by irritation from too-frequent rubbing, by prolonged exposure to dry, smoky air or chlorinated swimming-pool water, or by the consumption of alcohol. Rest and try to remove or avoid the suspected offending agents—smoke, chlorine and the like—and use any over-the-counter eye drops that soothe your eyes. However, if other symptoms occur with eye redness, or if redness seems excessive or chronic, see a doctor.

● **Red eyes often are accompanied by excess secretions** on the surface of the eye. Such secretions can cause temporary blurring of vision, which usually can be relieved by blinking. The type of secretion may suggest the cause of the redness.

If red, irritated eyes are accompanied by a thick, sticky discharge that causes the eyelids to stick together, the problem may be BACTERIAL CONJUNCTIVITIS, a bacterial infection of the undersides of the eyelids and the whites of the eyes. Often called pinkeye, this infection easily spreads from one eye to the other, as well as to other people. Consult a physician within a few days.

If red eyes are accompanied by a profuse watery discharge, the cause may be VIRAL CONJUNCTIVITIS, a viral infection of the undersides of the eyelids and the whites of the eyes. An upper-respiratory infection may have preceded the ailment, and you may note the presence of swollen lymph glands at the outer edge of the cheek, just in front of the ear. The inner aspect of the eyelids may show numerous small raised bumps. Consult a physician within 24 hours.

If red eyes are accompanied by pronounced itching and watering, the cause may be ALLERGIC CONJUNCTIVITIS, sensitivity of the undersides of the eyelids and the whites of the eyes to pollen or chemicals such as are found in hair spray and eye make-up. Avoid suspected agents, take antihistamines and consult a physician if symptoms are severe or persistent.

● **Red eyes that are accompanied by either marked eye pain or extraordinary visual impairment** suggest a disorder requiring prompt treatment.

If a red, painful eye occurs suddenly with decreased or blurred vision, the cause may be ACUTE GLAUCOMA, increased pressure on the retina due to excess fluid in the eye. Nausea and vomiting may also be present. Consult a physician immediately.

If a red, painful eye occurs suddenly with blurred vision, painful sensitivity to light or pain on moving the eye, the problem may be either KERATITIS, infection of the cornea, or UVEITIS, infection of the iris. Consult a physician immediately.

• **One dramatic cause of eye redness—often more alarming than dangerous**—is HYPHEMA, bleeding into the white portion of the eye. It can be caused by a scratch from a fingernail or a blow to the eye, but it can also occur spontaneously after a sneeze or cough. If there is no visual impairment or pain, you can wait for several hours to see the doctor, but consult a physician immediately if there is any change in vision or if there is any chance that foreign material has lodged in the eye.

RINGING IN THE EARS. Ringing in the ears, TINNITUS, can be a buzzing, whistling, hissing or roaring sound as well as bell-like. It can be heard in one or both ears, and is more frequently noticed at night, when background noises decrease. Ringing may be a side effect of many common drugs, it may follow exposure to loud noises such as a gunshot or loud music, and it is a common consequence of aging. But ringing is also a symptom of many ear disorders, some minor and transient but others serious. If ringing persists after the most obvious causes have been eliminated, get a thorough ear examination; this is especially true if ringing is confined to one ear or is associated with hearing loss or dizziness.

• **Ringing in the ears that follows use of certain drugs** may be caused by them. The principal offenders are aspirin in large doses, the heart medicine quinidine, the malaria drug quinine (even the quinine water used to mix a gin and tonic), and the antibiotic streptomycin. If you must take these drugs on a regular basis, consult a physician at the first sign of ringing.

• **Ringing in the ears can suggest any of several ear ailments.** In such cases, the hearing changes usually are accompanied by other symptoms that provide the clues to the ailment's origin.

If ringing and fullness in one ear are associated with hearing loss, the cause may be a blockage (see CLOGGED EARS) from impacted wax or an infection. Unless the ringing can be eliminated simply by removing wax, consult a physician within a few hours.

If ringing in one ear is associated with hearing loss and mild dizziness, the cause may be ACOUSTIC NEUROMA, a tumor on the nerve to the ear. Consult a physician within a day or two.

If ringing and fullness in one ear are associated with hearing loss, headache and repeated attacks of severely disabling dizziness, the cause may be MÉNIÈRE'S DISEASE, a disorder of the inner ear that primarily affects middle-aged men. The attacks of dizzi-

ness, called vertigo, are often described as a severe whirling phenomenon in which the room spins to such a degree that nausea, vomiting and profuse sweating also occur. Consult a physician within several days if symptoms pass quickly, sooner if they are severe or persistent.

SENSITIVITY TO LIGHT. Sudden exposure to bright light normally causes discomfort. When such pain is continuous, it is called photophobia, literally, "fear of light." Mild degrees of photophobia often are associated with such ailments as INFLUENZA, TENSION HEADACHE and MIGRAINE HEADACHE. For temporary, mild episodes of light sensitivity, you should rest, remain in a dimly lit room and take aspirin. Wear sunglasses if necessary. Severe or persistent uncomfortable sensitivity to light is another matter and demands medical attention.

If severely painful sensitivity to light occurs suddenly, without ready explanation, or if it follows shortly after you have had a foreign object in your eye, it may indicate a serious disorder such as KERATITIS, an inflamed or infected cornea, or UVEITIS, an inflamed or infected iris. Consult a physician immediately.

If painful sensitivity to light follows exposure to ultraviolet light—usually from sunlamps, welding torches or sunlight reflected off snow or water—the cause may be ULTRAVIOLET KERATITIS, inflammation of the cornea by ultraviolet rays. This condition is commonly called SNOW BLINDNESS. There may be excess watering of the eye or a sensation of grit, sand or a foreign body in the eye. Medical treatment can ease discomfort but cannot speed healing, which should occur within two or three days.

If an infant exhibits marked sensitivity to light and has persistently closed eyelids as well as a watery or tear-filled eye, these symptoms may suggest INFANTILE GLAUCOMA, a disease marked by increased pressure inside the eyeball due to excess fluid. Consult a physician immediately.

SMELLING DIFFICULTY. Decreased ability to smell is usually caused by nasal congestion, but it can also occur after head injury or following an attack of INFLUENZA.

If smelling difficulty accompanies a common cold or an allergy, it is probably a side effect of nasal congestion. Use decongestants, antihistamine tablets or any over-the-counter nasal sprays to reduce such congestion; do not use these products for more than one week without consulting a doctor.

If loss of smell is associated with chronic nasal congestion and with a persistent nasal tone to the voice, it may indicate NASAL POLYPS, enlarged or swollen tissues in the nose. Consult a physician if symptoms are bothersome.

SNOW BLINDNESS. *See SENSITIVITY TO LIGHT*

SPOTS BEFORE THE EYES. Spots, stars or flashes of light usually are due to a bump on the head and need not cause concern unless there is persistently disturbed vision, bleeding in the eye or loss of consciousness. Another generally trivial phenomenon is floating spots, sometimes likened to dust particles drifting across the visual field. Such "floaters" are caused by loose tissue or bits of blood that sometimes get into eye fluids. Only if floaters occur more and more often or if any loss of vision occurs is medical help needed.

If a sudden shower of floaters passes before the eyes, or if spots recur with increasing frequency and are then followed, possibly after a few days, by a sudden loss of vision in one eye, the problem may be a RETINAL DETACHMENT, a partial or complete separation of the retina from the back of the eye. The visual loss is most often described as a shadow or curtain being drawn across the eye. Get medical attention immediately.

● **Halos around bright lights** can be caused by excess secretions on the surface of the eye. In such cases, vision generally will clear as the secretions are wiped away by blinking. If the eye is also red, it may suggest CONJUNCTIVITIS, an inflammation of the undersides of the eyelids and the whites of the eyes, sometimes called pinkeye. Consult a physician within a few days.

If halos do not clear on blinking and are accompanied by sudden blurred vision and severe eye pain and redness, the cause may be ACUTE GLAUCOMA, increased pressure on the retina due to excess fluid. There may also be severe nausea and vomiting. Consult a physician immediately. If such halos occur without eye pain, but with blurred or dimmed vision, CHRONIC GLAUCOMA may be the cause. Consult a physician within a day or two.

If halos around lights develop gradually and seem to be worse at night, they may indicate a CATARACT, a clouding of the lens. This correctable condition occurs primarily in elderly individuals. Consult a physician within several days.

● **Flashing lights, bright zigzag lines or small blind spots that afflict one eye, occur suddenly** and pass within half an hour, only to be replaced by throbbing pain on one side of the head, may suggest CLASSIC MIGRAINE HEADACHE, caused by narrowed and then dilated blood vessels supplying the eyes and brain. Head pain may last for several hours and be accompanied by nausea, vomiting and sensitivity to light. If vision returns to normal and head pain passes, you can wait to see the doctor; but if symptoms persist or worsen, consult a physician within a few hours.

TASTE CHANGES. The ability to taste is lessened by use of tobacco, alcohol and, for some flavors, iced foods. Changes in tasting ability can accompany congestion from a COMMON COLD or an allergy; a nonprescription decongestant or antihistamine may help. Changes in the sense of taste can also occur during pregnancy, after a head injury, following a bout of INFLUENZA, or as a side effect of CANCER CHEMOTHERAPY. However, the symptom, if it is persistent, can point to the existence of serious disease and should be called to a doctor's attention.

● **Changes in taste that occur suddenly and are accompanied by cough, headache, fatigue, joint pain or the yellow skin of jaundice** may suggest HEPATITIS, an inflamed liver. Consult a physician within 24 hours. One particularly common experience is a sudden aversion for the taste of cigarettes.

TINGLING. *See TOUCH CHANGES*

TOUCH CHANGES. The ability to sense pain, pressure, vibration, temperature and position can be affected by drug and alcohol use and by a variety of medical conditions—some serious, most not. Some interfere with ability to detect pain; others with the sense of where an arm or leg is in space; still others with all of the sensations that, taken together, form the sense of touch. A person experiencing a change in the sense of touch may feel burning sensations, numbness or tingling, or may feel nothing at all. Reasons for the change may be obvious enough: A burn or cut may heal over with scar tissue, leaving the affected area basically without touch receptors. But because some changes in the sense of touch can signal serious diseases or injuries of the brain, spinal cord and nerves, you should consult a physician if any interruption of touch is persistent or unduly unpleasant.

● **Numbness, burning or tingling feelings in an arm or leg** may suggest that the limb is "asleep"—that is, its circulation has been cut off temporarily, robbing nerves and tissues of blood. This common occurrence almost always is the result of maintaining one position for too long. Its cure is simple: Change positions.

● **Numbness, burning or tingling feelings in the hand, wrist or forearm that follow a bump to the elbow** almost always signal a jarring of the ULNAR NERVE, the nerve that lies just beneath the skin near the inner knob of the elbow. Hitting this "funny bone" is an unpleasant and frequently painful sensation. There is little you can do about it except rub and wait for the pain to pass.

If numbness, burning or tingling feelings in the hand, fingers, wrist or forearm occur seemingly without cause, the problem may be CARPAL TUNNEL SYNDROME, pressure on a nerve in the wrist. The pressure may result from inflammation of a tendon or from arthritis. The condition mainly affects middle-aged women and usually disappears, without treatment, in a few months. Consult a physician if symptoms are bothersome.

TUNNEL VISION. People vary in their ability to see objects at the edges of the field of view. This is normal. What is not normal is the restriction of sight to a narrow area at the center of view, as if everything were seen through a cardboard tube. Such tunnel vision in many cases develops gradually, in one eye or both. This gradual onset often keeps the problem from being noticed; it pays to watch for it, because this symptom can suggest a serious eye disorder that can be treated successfully if caught in its early stages but may cause blindness if neglected.

● **Gradual loss of peripheral vision, or slowly constricting tunnel vision, that occurs in a person over 40** may suggest CHRONIC GLAUCOMA, a disorder characterized by a gradual rise in eyeball pressure. Although peripheral vision is the first to suffer, the elevated eyeball pressure eventually can damage or destroy central sight. Be particularly wary of this disorder if relatives have had it; chronic glaucoma runs in families. Consult a physician at the first sign of loss of peripheral vision.

UNCOORDINATED EYES. Eyes that do not work together—that fail, for example, to converge on close objects—are more noticeable to others than to the victim; the eyes seem to cross or to diverge sideways (walleyes) or vertically (hypertropia). The condition can result from brain or nerve disease or from injury to the eye or head. More often, however, it suggests a chronic disorder of the muscles that control eye movement.

● **Eyes that turn abnormally inward, outward or upward,** either at the same time or independently of each other, usually suggest STRABISMUS, an imbalance in muscles controlling eye movement. Double vision may occur, and it may be constant or intermittent. Strabismus can be present at birth, but more often it develops in childhood. Consult a physician; if neglected, the disorder can destroy sight in one eye. Special glasses and eye exercises often solve the problem, but in many cases surgery is needed.

● **Eyes that oscillate uncontrollably,** moving back and forth or up and down, suggest NYSTAGMUS, a motor disorder that can be present at birth, the result of brain or nerve disease; alcohol or drugs can also cause it. In the most common form of the disorder, JERK NYSTAGMUS, the eye may drift away from the object of focus, then jerk back. Vision may be blurred. Consult a physician within a day or so.

VISION LOSS. *See BLURRED VISION, CLOUDY VISION, COLOR BLINDNESS, DIMMING VISION, DOUBLE VISION, NIGHT BLINDNESS, SPOTS BEFORE THE EYES, TUNNEL VISION*

WALLEYES. *See UNCOORDINATED EYES*

Bibliography

BOOKS

Abrahamson, Ira A., *Know Your Eyes*. Krieger, 1977.

Adams, George L., et al., *Boies's Fundamentals of Otolaryngology*. W. B. Saunders, 1978.

Albe-Fessard, D., et al., *Handbook of Sensory Physiology,* Vol. II. Springer-Verlag, 1973.

Asimov, Isaac, *The Human Brain: Its Capacities and Functions*. Houghton Mifflin, 1964.

Baker, Jeffrey, *The Truth About Contact Lenses: Everything the Wearer, or Potential Wearer, Should Know*. G. P. Putnam's Sons, 1970.

Ballenger, John Jacob, *Diseases of the Nose, Throat and Ear*. Lea & Febiger, 1977.

Bedichek, Roy, *The Sense of Smell*. Doubleday, 1960.

Carterette, Edward C., and Morton P. Friedman, *Handbook of Perception*. Academic, 1978.

Chalkley, Thomas, *Your Eyes*. Charles C. Thomas, 1974.

Cogniat, Raymond, *Monet and His World*. Transl. by Wayne Dynes. London: Thames and Hudson, 1966.

DeWeese, David D., *Textbook of Otolaryngology*. C. V. Mosby, 1982.

Duane, Thomas D., ed., *Clinical Ophthalmology,* Vol. 5. Harper & Row, 1981.

Eden, John, *The Eye Book*. Viking, 1978.

Esterman, Ben, *The Eye Book: A Specialist's Guide to Your Eyes and Their Care*. Great Ocean, 1977.

Freese, Arthur S., *The Miracle of Vision*. Harper & Row, 1977.
You and Your Hearing: How to Protect It, Preserve It, and Restore It. Charles Scribner's Sons, 1979.

Goodhill, Victor, *Ear Diseases, Deafness, and Dizziness*. Harper & Row, 1979.

Griffin, Donald R., *Echoes of Bats and Men*. Doubleday, 1959.

Handbook of Nonprescription Drugs. American Pharmaceutical Association, 1979.

Helleberg, Marilyn M., *Your Hearing Loss: How to Break the Sound Barrier*. Nelson-Hall, 1979.

Hunt, C. C., ed., *Neurophysiology*. University Park, 1975.

Johnson, G. Timothy, and Stephen E. Goldfinger, eds., *The Harvard Medical School Health Letter Book*. Harvard University Press, 1981.

Kaplan, Harold I., et al., *Comprehensive Textbook of Psychiatry,* Vol. 3. Williams & Wilkins, 1980.

Keefe, Robert J., *I Care: Eye Care at Work, Home and Play*. Physicians Art Services, 1979.

Keen, Harry, et al., eds., *Triumphs of Medicine*. Paul Elek, 1976.

Keller, Helen Adams, *Helen Keller in Scotland*. London: Methuen, 1933.

Labaree, Leonard W., ed., *The Papers of Benjamin Franklin*. Yale University Press, 1961.

Masterton, R. Bruce, ed., *Handbook of Behavioral Neurobiology,* Vol. 1. Plenum, 1978.

Miller, David, *Ophthalmology: The Essentials*. Houghton Mifflin, 1979.

Milne, Lorus, and Margery Milne, *The Senses of Animals and Men*. Atheneum, 1962.

Mindel, Eugene D., and McCay Vernon, *They Grow in Silence—The Deaf Child and His Family*. National Association of the Deaf, 1971.

Montagu, Ashley, *Touching: The Human Significance of the Skin*. Columbia University Press, 1971.

Morrison, Robert J., *The Contact Lens Book*. Human Research Laboratories Publishing Corporation, 1976.

Newell, Frank W., and J. Terry Ernest, *Ophthalmology: Principles and Concepts*. C. V. Mosby, 1974.

New Orleans Academy of Ophthalmology, *Symposium on Medical and Surgical Diseases of the Cornea*. C. V. Mosby, 1980.
Symposium on Retina and Retinal Surgery. C. V. Mosby, 1969.

Nilsson, Lennart, *Behold Man: A Photographic Journey of Discovery Inside the Body*. Little, Brown, 1973.

Northern, Jerry L., ed., *Hearing Disorders*. Little, Brown, 1976.

Paparella, Michael M., and Donald A. Shumrick, eds., *Otolaryngology,* Vols. 1 and 2. W. B. Saunders, 1973.

Rosenberg, Mark L., *Patients: The Experience of Illness*. W. B. Saunders, 1980.

Roueché, Berton, *The Medical Detectives*. Washington Square, 1980.

Saunders, William H., et al., *Nursing Care in Eye, Ear, Nose, and Throat Disorders*. C. V. Mosby, 1979.

Scheie, Harold G., and Daniel M. Albert, *Textbook of Ophthalmology*. W. B. Saunders, 1977.

Sloane, Albert E., *So You Have Cataracts: What You and Your Family Should Know*. Charles C. Thomas, 1970.

Stein, Harold A., and Bernard J. Slatt, *The Ophthalmic Assistant: Fundamentals and Clinical Practice*. C. V. Mosby, 1976.

Trevor-Roper, P. D., *Lecture Notes on Ophthalmology*. Oxford: Blackwell Scientific Publications, 1974.

Trevor-Roper, P. D., ed., *Recent Advances in Ophthalmology*. Churchill Livingstone, 1975.

Vaughan, Daniel, and Taylor Asbury, *General Ophthalmology*. Lange Medical Publications, 1980.

Veirs, Everett R., *So You Have Glaucoma*. Grune & Stratton, 1970.

Zinn, Walter J., and Herbert Solomon, *The Complete Guide to Eye Care, Eyeglasses and Contact Lenses*. Frederick Fell, 1977.

PERIODICALS

Avery, Caryl S., ''Your Ears: A Caring, Kissing, Flirting, Shaping, Balancing Guide to Their Total Health and Beauty.'' *Self,* July 1981.

Bartoshuk, Linda, ''Separate Worlds of Taste.'' *Psychology Today,* September 1980.

Bohne, Barbara A., et al., ''Rock Music and Inner Ear Damage.'' *American Family Physician,* May 1977.

Brackman, Derald E., and Robert G. Anderson, ''Ménière's Disease: Treatment Strategies and Results of the Endolymphatic Subarachnoid Shunt in 125 Cases.'' *Otolaryngologic Clinics of North America,* Vol. 13, No. 4, November 1980.

Cain, William S., ''Educating Your Nose.'' *Psychology Today,* July, 1981.

''Controversial Research into New Kind of Sight.'' *Medical World News,* September 5, 1969.

Dobelle, W. H., and M. G. Mladejovsky, ''Artificial Vision for the Blind: Electrical Stimulation of Visual Cortex Offers Hope for a Functional Prosthesis.'' *Science,* Vol. 183, February 1974.

Dobelle, W. H., et al., '' 'Braille' Reading by a Blind Volunteer by Visual Cortex Stimulation.'' *Nature,* Vol. 259, January 15, 1976.

Doty, Richard L., ''A Review of Olfactory Dysfunctions in Man.'' *American Journal of Otolaryngology,* Vol. 1, No. 1, Fall 1979.

Dunkle, Terry, ''The Sound of Silence.'' *Science 82,* April 1982.

Freeman, H. MacKenzie, ''Recent Advances in Retinal Detachment and Vitreous Surgery.'' *Association of Operating Room Nurses Journal,* Vol. 18, No. 5, November 1973.

Hahn, H., ''Über die Ursache der Geschmacks-Empfindung.'' *Klinische Wochenschrift,* Vol. 15, 1936.

Hopson, Janet L., ''Scent and Human Behavior: Olfaction or Fiction?'' *Science News*, Vol. 115, April 28, 1979.

''Intraocular Lens Implantation.'' *NIH Consensus Development Conference Summary*, Vol. 2, No. 7, September 10-11, 1979.

Kurzweil, Raymond, ''Giving 'Sight' to the Blind.'' *SciQuest*, February 1981.

Mason, Allen, and John Pratt, ''Touch.'' *Nursing Times*, June 5, 1980.

Massler, Maury, ''Geriatric Nutrition: The Role of Taste and Smell in Appetite.'' *The Journal of Prosthetic Dentistry*, Vol. 43, No. 3, March 1980.

Michelson, Robin P., ''Multichannel Cochlear Implants.'' *Otolaryngologic Clinics of North America*, Vol. 11, No. 1, February 1978.

''Olfactory Synchrony of Menstrual Cycles.'' *Science News*, July 2, 1977.

Paton, David, and John A. Craig, ''Cataracts: Development, Diagnosis, and Management.'' *Clinical Symposia*, Vol. 26, No. 3, 1974.

Perham, Chris, ''The Sound of Silence.'' *EPA Journal*, October 1979.

Schiffman, Susan, and Marcy Pasternak, ''Decreased Discrimination of Food Odors in the Elderly.'' *Journal of Gerontology*, Vol. 34, No. 1, 1979.

Treisman, Michel, ''Motion Sickness: An Evolutionary Hypothesis.'' *Science*, Vol. 197, July 1977.

Weiss, Sandra J., ''The Language of Touch.'' *Nursing Research*, March-April 1979.

''Will Surgery on the Cornea Render Spectacles Obsolete?'' *Journal of the American Medical Association*, Vol. 245, No. 9, March 6, 1981.

OTHER PUBLICATIONS

''Contact Lens News Backgrounder.'' American Optometric Association, April 1981.

''Eye Wear Then and Now News Backgrounder.'' American Optometric Association, May 1981.

''Facts and Figures.'' National Society to Prevent Blindness, 1980.

''The Fifth National Science Writers Seminar in Ophthalmology.'' Research to Prevent Blindness, Inc., May 8-11, 1976.

Mellor, C. Michael, ed., ''Aids for the 80s: What They Are and What They Do.'' American Foundation for the Blind, 1981.

''Vision Research: A National Plan: 1978-1982,'' Vol. 2. U.S. Department of Health, Education, and Welfare, 1977.

Picture credits

The sources for the illustrations that appear in this book are listed below. Credits for the illustrations from left to right are separated by semicolons, from top to bottom by dashes.

Cover: Enrico Ferorelli. 7: Fil Hunter. 9: Drawing by Cynthia Richardson. 11: © 1980 John Neubauer. 15-17: Nick Barrington, Axbridge, England. 20: Lee Lockwood. 22: CIBA Pharmaceutical Company. 24-32: © 1974 Lennart Nilsson from *Behold Man*, Little, Brown and Co. Drawings by Joan McGurren. 33: Drawing from the Studio of Kathryn D. Rebeiz—© 1974 Lennart Nilsson, from *Behold Man*, Little, Brown and Co. 34, 35: Drawing by Cynthia Richardson; © 1974 Lennart Nilsson, from *Behold Man*, Little, Brown and Co. 37: David Sharpe. 38: Courtesy of Perkins School for the Blind. 40: Drawing by Cynthia Richardson. 44: Aldo Tutino—Drawings by Cynthia Richardson. 46: Robert S. Preston, courtesy Professor J. E. Hawkins, Kresge Hearing Research Institute, Univ. of Michigan Medical School. 48: Adapted from R. Hull, ''Hearing Evaluation of the Elderly.'' In J. Katz (Ed.) *Handbook of Clinical Audiology*, Second Edition. Baltimore: Williams & Wilkins Co., 1978. 50-61: Linda Bartlett. 63: Dan McCoy from Rainbow. 66, 67: Frederic F. Bigio from B-C Graphics. 71-74: Richard Anderson. 76: The Beck Engraving Company. 78, 79: American Optical Corporation. 81: © 1981 Ted Kawalerski from The Image Bank. 82-85: Fil Hunter. Drawings from the Studio of Kathryn D. Rebeiz. 87: William C. Nyberg RBP. 91: Barrett P. Walker. 92: Hank Morgan from Rainbow. 95: Arthur O'Neill, photographer, The Carroll Center for the Blind. 96, 97: Fil Hunter, courtesy Volunteers for the Visually Handicapped, Bethesda. 98-107: © Gordon Baer, Cincinnati. 109: Ron Campise, House Ear Institute. 111: © Alexander Tsiaras. 112, 113: Dan McCoy from Rainbow. 115: Frederic F. Bigio from B-C Graphics; Mark L. Rosenberg, M.D., from *Patients: The Experience of Illness*, © 1980 by W. B. Saunders Company. 116-118: Mark L. Rosenberg, M.D., from *Patients: The Experience of Illness*, © 1980 by W. B. Saunders Company. Drawing from the Studio of Kathryn D. Rebeiz. 120: Csaba L. Martonyi, The Univ. of Michigan. 122: Walter Hilmers Jr. from HJ Commercial Art; NASA. 124, 125: Dan McCoy from Rainbow. Drawing by Frederic F. Bigio from B-C Graphics. 126-135: © Alexander Tsiaras. Drawings from the Studio of Kathryn D. Rebeiz. 137: David Sharpe, courtesy of Designs for Living, Inc. 138: © 1981 Erich Lessing, Kunst-Und Kulturarchiv, Vienna. 141: Green and Hahn Photography Ltd., Christchurch, New Zealand. 143: Lee Lockwood. 144: Frederic F. Bigio from B-C Graphics. 145: House Ear Institute. 146-155: Lee Lockwood.

Acknowledgments

The index for this book was prepared by Barbara L. Klein. For their help with this volume, the editors wish to thank the following: Karen S. Berliner, House Ear Institute, Los Angeles; Dr. Alex Bouteneff, Johns Hopkins Univ. Hospital, Baltimore; Dr. Richard Brilliant, Pennsylvania College of Optometry, Philadelphia; Mary Brink, South Kent, Conn.; Dr. Richard M. Chavis, Washington, D.C.; William W. Clark, Central Institute for the Deaf, St. Louis; Carter Collins, Smith Kettlewell Institute of Visual Sciences, San Francisco; Dr. Ziad E. Deeb, Washington Hospital Center, Washington, D.C.; Dr. Hugh de Fries, Washington Hospital Center, Washington, D.C.; Mr. and Mrs. Gordon Edwards, Cincinnati; Richard Evenson, National Library Service for the Blind and Physically Handicapped, Washington, D.C.; Joan Fergerson, Kendall Demonstration Elementary School, Washington, D.C.; Leslie Kay, Univ. of Canterbury, Christchurch, New Zealand; Dr. Charles Kelman, New York City; Hiroshi Kohno, Kanehara and Company, Ltd., Tokyo; Paul Lighty, Lafayette, N.J.; John Linvill, Stanford Univ. School of Engineering, Palo Alto, Calif.; Dr. Jerald J. Littlefield, Alexandria, Va.; Csaba L. Martonyi, Univ. of Michigan, Ann Arbor; Dr. R. Bruce Masterton, Florida State Univ., Tallahassee; Dr. Ronald Michels, Johns Hopkins Univ. Hospital, Baltimore; National Eye Institute, Bethesda, Md.; Arthur O'Neill, Carroll Center for the Blind, Newton, Mass.; Dr. Edward R. Perl, Univ. of North Carolina, Chapel Hill; Dr. Robert Petersen, Children's Hospital, Boston; Dr. Leonard J. Press, The Eye Institute Pediatric Unit, Philadelphia; Charlotte Rancilio, American Optometric Association, St. Louis; Dr. Ross Roeser, Dallas; Royal Commonwealth Society for the Blind, Sussex, England; Sensory Aids Corporation, Bensenville, Ill.; Dr. Norman Stahl, Bellmore, N.Y.; Alex Townsend, American Foundation for the Blind, New York City; Raymond Triebert, American School for the Deaf, West Hartford, Conn.; Hubert W. Upton, Arlington, Tex.; Volunteers for the Visually Handicapped, Bethesda, Md.; Dr. Richard Wender, New York City; Ed Zilberts, House Ear Institute, Los Angeles; George Zimmerman, Boston College, Chestnut Hill, Mass.

Index